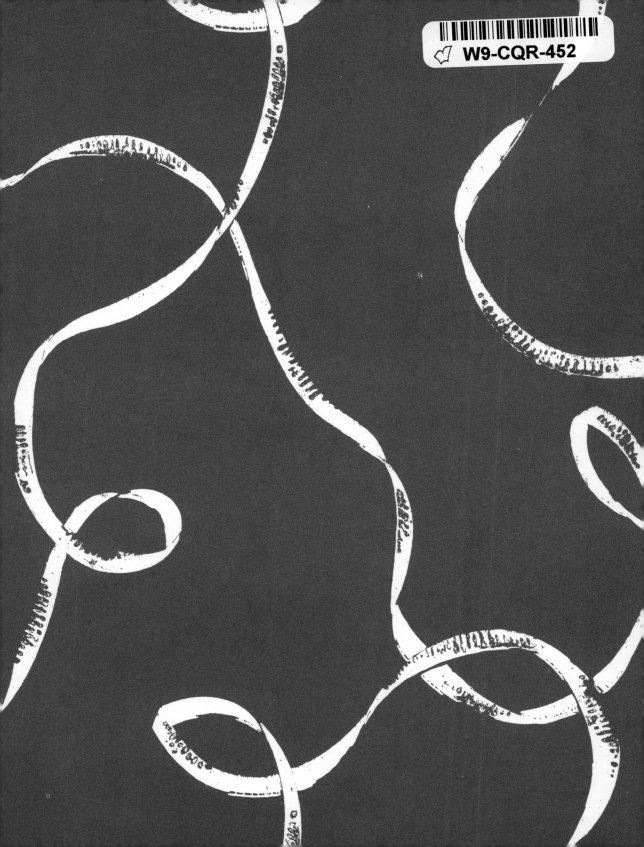

Impressions

A Palette of Fine Memphis Dining

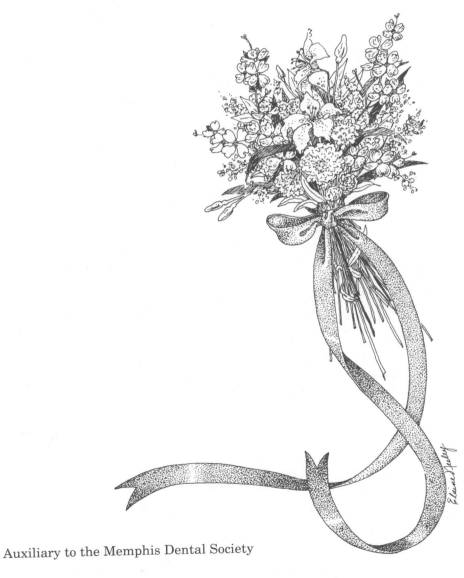

Auxiliary to the Memphis Dental Society

Copies of *Impressions* may be obtained by sending a check

for $16.95 plus $2.50 mailing cost
(Tennessee residents add $1.31 for sales tax) to:

P.O. Box 17272
Memphis, Tennessee 38187-0272

First printing   October, 1990   5,000 copies
Second printing   November, 1991   5,000 copies
Library of Congress Catalog Card Number 90-91626
ISBN 0-9626242-0-9

Copyright 1990 by
Auxiliary to the Memphis Dental Society

Cover design and illustrations by Elaine Speed Neeley

This book contains favorite recipes of members of the Auxiliary to the Memphis Dental Society and their friends. We do not claim that all recipes are original, only that they are our favorites. We regret that we were unable to include many recipes which were submitted due to similarity or lack of space. A special thank you to our members who gave unselfishly of their time and to our families who have been so patient and supportive during the past three years.

Printed in the USA by
WIMMER BROTHERS
A Wimmer Company
Memphis • Dallas

Introduction

Impressions are vivid remembrances. Each family within the Memphis dental community has its own treasured traditions of celebration for the special moments in their lives.

Eating is a ritual on holidays, family days and every day. This book presents the ways we come together with family and friends for a few precious moments. Like the brief life of a flower, these moments are never long enough, so we try to extend these times with a little extra care and love; each recipe in this book has been tested and retested with that same care and love.

We are delighted to be able to bring you our ideas for creating new and lasting *Impressions* in your life.

We dedicate this book to

Bettye Hudson

(Mrs. Frank J.)

who exemplifies the spirit of voluntarism which exists throughout the Memphis dental community. Bettye, a loyal, loving and devoted member of our Auxiliary for over 35 years, has served as President of the Auxiliary to the Memphis Dental Society and as President of the Auxiliary to the Tennessee Dental Association. Our resident chef, Bettye, always has one gracious smile and two willing hands.

For over half a century, the Memphis community has benefited from the contributions of the auxiliary, both in financial aid and volunteer hours. Funding for dental clinics in hospitals, treatment centers and care homes is an ongoing concern. The elderly, as well as the young, have benefited from the distribution of hundreds of thousands of toothbrush kits; Teddy, the Tooth and Merry Mary the Clown, continue to communicate the need for good dental health in nursing homes and schools. Through a major contribution of the auxiliary to the Health Science Wing of the Memphis Pink Palace Museum, the history of dentistry in the south has been preserved for future generations.

Proceeds from the sale of *Impressions* will be returned to the Memphis community for the continuation of these and other dental related projects.

Golden Patron
The Memphis Dental Society

Silver Patron
University of Tennessee College of Dentistry

Patrons

Dr. and Mrs. William K. Barrett, III
Dr. and Mrs. John Mallett Barron
Mrs. James F. Bennett, Jr.
Dr. and Mrs. James F. Bigger, Jr.
Dr. and Mrs. Lesley H. Binkley, Jr.
Dr. and Mrs. George H. Bouldien
Dr. and Mrs. J. Roy Bourgoyne
Dr. and Mrs. W. L. Burgess, Jr.
Dr. and Mrs. Kenneth M. Caldwell
Dr. and Mrs. J. Thomas Cobb
Dr. and Mrs. James B. Cochran
Dr. and Mrs. William O. Coley, Jr.
Dr. and Mrs. Phillip O. Dowdle
Dr. W. David Edmonds
Mrs. A. Joe Fuson
Dr. and Mrs. Joseph W. Graham
Dr. and Mrs. Charles E. Harbison
Dr. and Mrs. Sam H. Hardison
Dr. and Mrs. Richard C. Harris
Dr. and Mrs. Michael J. Harty
Dr. and Mrs. Fernando C. Heros
Dr. and Mrs. Jack W. Hoelscher
Dr. and Mrs. Frank J. Hudson
Dr. and Mrs. Tony Hughey
Mrs. O. M. Jamison
Dr. and Mrs. Charles B. Lansden
Dr. and Mrs. Warren L. Lesmeister
Dr. and Mrs. David R. Libby
Dr. and Mrs. Chester Lloyd
Dr. and Mrs. J. Howard McClain
Dr. and Mrs. Bruce H. McCullar
E. L. Mercere, Inc.
Dr. and Mrs. H. Franklin Miller
Dr. and Mrs. Preston D. Miller, Jr.

Dr. and Mrs. Joe Hall Morris
Dr. and Mrs. Lyle E. Muller
Dr. and Mrs. R. Malcolm Overbey
Dr. and Mrs. Robert L. Parrish, Jr.
Dr. and Mrs. William R. Priester, III
Dr. and Mrs. Thomas C. Pyron
Mrs. Robert H. Ramey
Dr. and Mrs. Richard J. Reynolds
Dr. and Mrs. Morris L. Robbins
Dr. and Mrs. James R. Ross
Dr. and Mrs. David K. Rowe
Dr. and Mrs. Walter Cooper Sandusky, Jr.
Dr. and Mrs. Walter Cooper Sandusky, III
Dr. and Mrs. James E. Sexton
Dr. and Mrs. Phillip Sherman, Jr.
Dr. and Mrs. T. H. Shipmon
Dr. and Mrs. O'Farrell Shoemaker
Dr. and Mrs. Ernest H. Sigman, Jr.
Dr. and Mrs. William F. Slagle
Dr. and Mrs. Roy M. Smith
Dr. and Mrs. James G. Sousoulas
Dr. and Mrs. Eugene O. Thomas
Dr. and Mrs. Harold P. Thomas
Dr. and Mrs. N. Edward Tillman
Dr. and Mrs. Justin D. Towner
Mrs. Buford F. Wallace
Dr. and Mrs. J. Stephen Weir
Dr. and Mrs. Edward J. Wiener
Dr. and Mrs. Charles E. Wilkinson
Dr. and Mrs. Gray Williams
Dr. and Mrs. Lee E. Wilson
Dr. and Mrs. John Winford, III
Dr. and Mrs. James L. Wiygul
Dr. and Mrs. Mark E. Wiygul

Memorials

Mrs. A. G. Baxter by Billie Jean Johnson
Dr. Ralph Waldo Handy by Sharolene Handy
Mrs. Zana Lee Jennings by Floy Mae Roser
Mrs. L. C. Templeton by Virginia Sullivan
Mrs. Kathryn Weber by Rose Marie Manning
Dr. Gray Williams by Elizabeth Williams

We sincerely thank these individuals for their generous contributions.

Chairmen

Mrs. Charles E. Harbison   Mrs. Phillip Sherman, Jr.

Manuscript Coordinator

Mrs. Preston D. Miller, Jr.

Committees

Steering Committee:
Mrs. John Mallett Barron
Mrs. Phillip O. Dowdle
Mrs. Charles E. Harbison
Mrs. Frank J. Hudson
Mrs. Tony Hughey
Mrs. Charles B. Lansden
Mrs. J. Howard McClain
Mrs. H. Franklin Miller
Mrs. Preston D. Miller, Jr.
Mrs. Phillip Sherman, Jr.

Recipe Collection:
Mrs. J. Garland Cherry
Mrs. Richard C. Harris
Mrs. Frank J. Hudson
Mrs. Joe Hall Morris
Mrs. Richard J. Reynolds

Recipe Testing:
Mrs. Michael J. Harty
Mrs. Jack W. Hoelscher
Mrs. James R. Ross
Mrs. William F. Slagle

Copywriting:
Mrs. John Mallett Barron
Mrs. H. Franklin Miller

Typing:
Mrs. James W. Breazeal
Mrs. Sam H. Hardison
Mrs. Trent G. Wilson
Mrs. Mark E. Wiygul
Mrs. E. Jack Wohrman, Jr.

Proofreading:
Mrs. James F. Bigger, Jr.
Mrs. J. Roy Bourgoyne
Mrs. Michael J. Harty
Mrs. Joe Hall Morris
Mrs. Ernest H. Sigman, Jr.
Mrs. James L. Wiygul

Promotion:
Mrs. Lesley H. Binkley, Jr.
Mrs. J. Stephen Weir

Marketing:
Mrs. Tony Hughey
Mrs. Stephen R. Maroda
Mrs. Bruce H. McCullar

Dental Society-Auxiliary Liaison:
Mrs. Joseph W. Graham

Art:
Mrs. William K. Barrett, III
Mrs. James F. Bennett, Jr.
Mrs. J. Thomas Cobb

Publicity:
Mrs. James E. Sexton

Finance:
Mrs. Sewell R. McKinney, C.P.A
Mrs. J. Howard McClain, Treasurer
Mrs. H. Franklin Miller, Contributions

Section Chairmen

Creative Entertaining
Mrs. John Mallett Barron
Mrs. H. Franklin Miller
Mrs. Justin D. Towner

Appetizers/Beverages
Mrs. Michael J. Harty

Soups/Salads
Mrs. John Cannon
Mrs. J. Lawrence McRae

Breads
Mrs. Preston D. Miller, Jr.
Mrs. Justin D. Towner

Brunches
Mrs. William F. Slagle

Entrées
Mrs. James F. Bennett, Jr.
Mrs. Lyle E. Muller
Mrs. James R. Ross

Vegetables and Side Dishes
Mrs. J. Roy Bourgoyne
Mrs. J. Stephen Weir

Desserts
Mrs. James F. Bennett, Jr.
Mrs. David R. Libby
Mrs. Richard C. Harris

Table of Contents

CREATIVE ENTERTAINING 9

APPETIZERS 33

BEVERAGES AND SOUPS 67

SALADS AND DRESSINGS 85

BREADS AND MUFFINS 115

ENTRÉES 145

    Meats 147

    Seafood 165

    Poultry 176

    Game 189

    Brunch 196

VEGETABLES AND SIDE DISHES 203

DESSERTS 231

    Pies 233

    Cakes 245

    Candies 260

    Cookies 265

    Desserts 273

About the Artist

Elaine Speed Neeley studied graphic design and art education at Memphis State University in Tennessee. In 1984, after teaching high school art for ten years, she established Hickory Ridge Studio in Memphis and began to concentrate on her own painting.

Born and raised in Nashville, Neeley has lived in Memphis since completing college. Her art includes a variety of subjects in different mediums such as oils, acrylics, pastels, pen and ink and watercolors. Her most recent works are of wildlife, florals, and city scenes of Memphis and Nashville.

Neeley is a member of the Memphis/Germantown Art League, and a volunteer for the Memphis Brooks Museum of Art Educational Outreach Program. In addition to her fine art, Neeley also does freelance graphic design and portraits, and continues to give private art instruction. Through both her own work and her teaching, she sees art as a means to provide others with an opportunity to really see and enjoy the beautiful things around them.

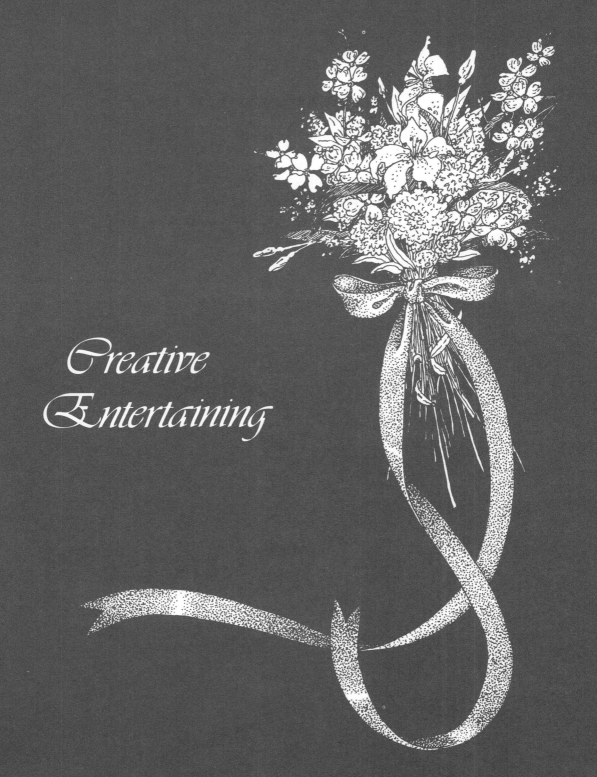

Creative
Entertaining

The Azaleas are Perfect

The azaleas are ablaze with fuchsia and pink, and the white dogwood blooms are fresh on the trees — a new beginning for everyone. Whether it's Passover, Easter or another Springtime holiday, this collage of traditional foods is a palate pleaser. The abundance of blossoms evident everywhere in Memphis in the Spring provides inspiration for decorating in profusion.

Spring Brunch

Mimosas

Stuffed Snow Peas 54

Oyster Crackers 59

Lamb Milanaise or Roasted Leg of Lamb 164, 163

Mint Sauce for Lamb 194

Fresh Asparagus

Baked Orange Glazed Carrots 210

Gazpacho Aspic with Marinated Artichoke Hearts 95

Pocketbook Rolls 133

Old Fashioned Strawberry Shortcake 301

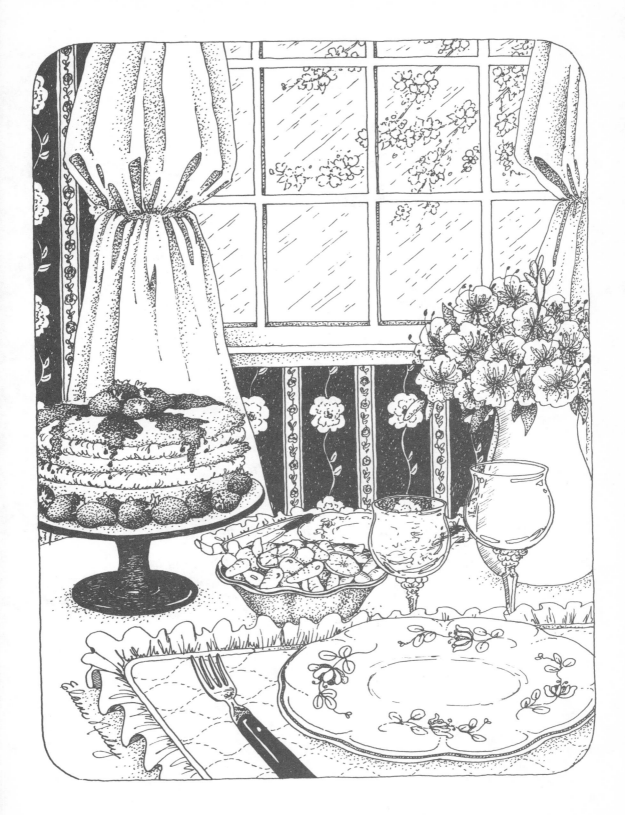

Congratulations and Accolades

In the dental family, no occasion is more important or worthy of celebration than "the" graduation. Naturally, only your very best table appointments will do, and a special place card for the honoree is a must. This menu will please the most exacting tastes for lunch or dinner.

Graduation Party

Gourmet Beef Tenderloin 148 with Béarnaise Sauce 192

Seafood with Wild Rice 170

Spinach Supreme 223

Avocado-Mandarin Green Salad 92

Vinaigrette Dressing or Poppy Seed Dressing 113

Jeanne Craddock's Rolls 132

Strawberry Jamaica 301

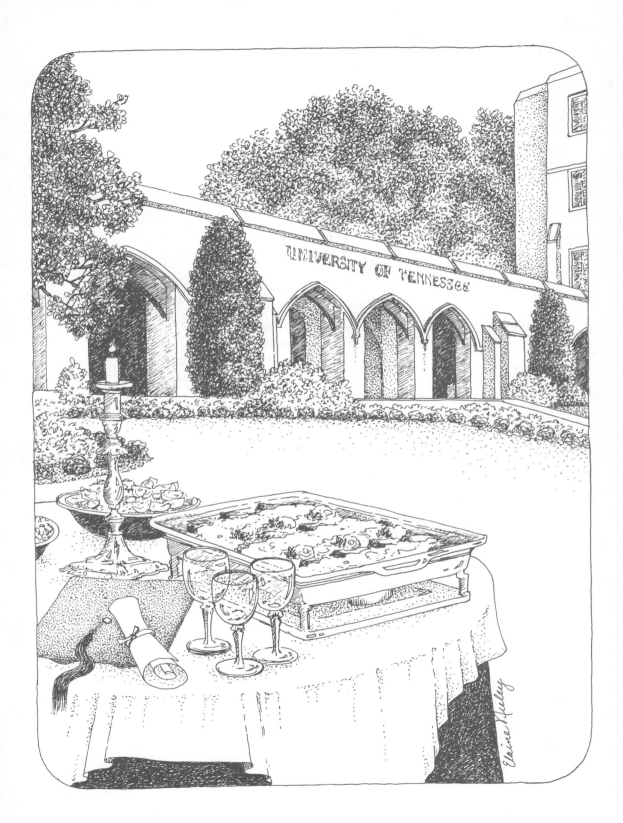

Ode to the Sunset

Each May, Memphians enjoy a glorious technicolor sunset at the annual Memphis in May Sunset Symphony. From dawn's early light, people gather at the river bluff to enjoy fun, food, and fellowship. When the strains of "Ole Man River", sung by the inimitable James Hyter, float over the crowd — the evening is complete.

Whether you choose Aunt Hattie's "wedding ring" quilt or color coordinated linens, your picnic hamper is spread in style. Don't forget to bring large coolers filled with ice.

Symphony Picnic on the River

Cream Vichyssoise 84

Crabmeat Pâté 52

Eye of Round on Ann's Dill Bread 149, 134

Horseradish Sauce

Artichoke and Rice Salad 102

Caramel Tennessee Bars 284

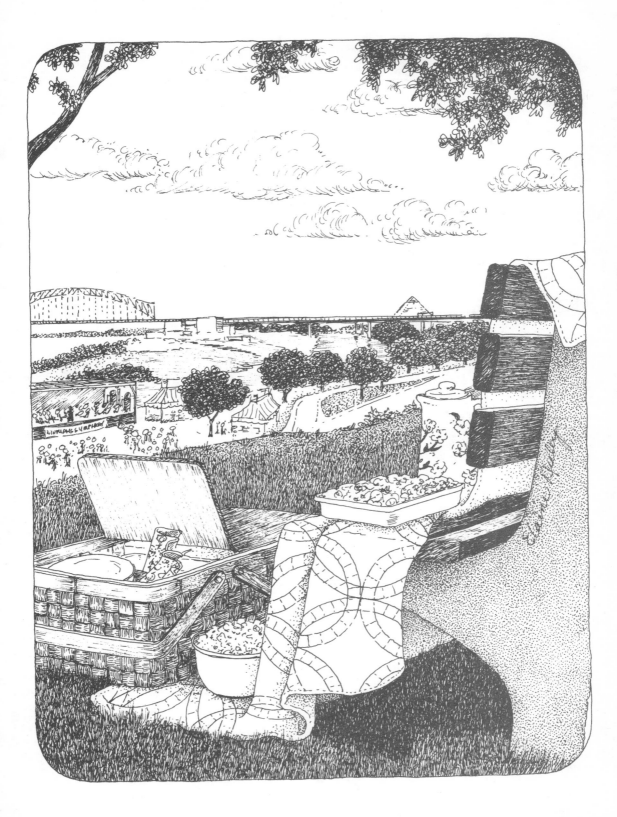

Mexican Wedding Party

It's your time to entertain for your favorite bride. We always think poolside for the summer. The taste of a fruity, cold sangría conjures up the idea of a Mexican Wedding Party al fresco. Think South-of-the-Border bright with piñatas, streamers, tin reflectors and the colors orange, red, purple, and turquoise. The recipes in this menu are some of the most requested of our hostesses.

Poolside Supper

Cheese Wafers 43

Mexican Tuna Dip 65

Gazpacho 79

Chicken Enchilada Casserole 178

Avocado Mousse 36

Bread Sticks

Pralines 269

Flan 294

Sangría 73

Mexican Beer

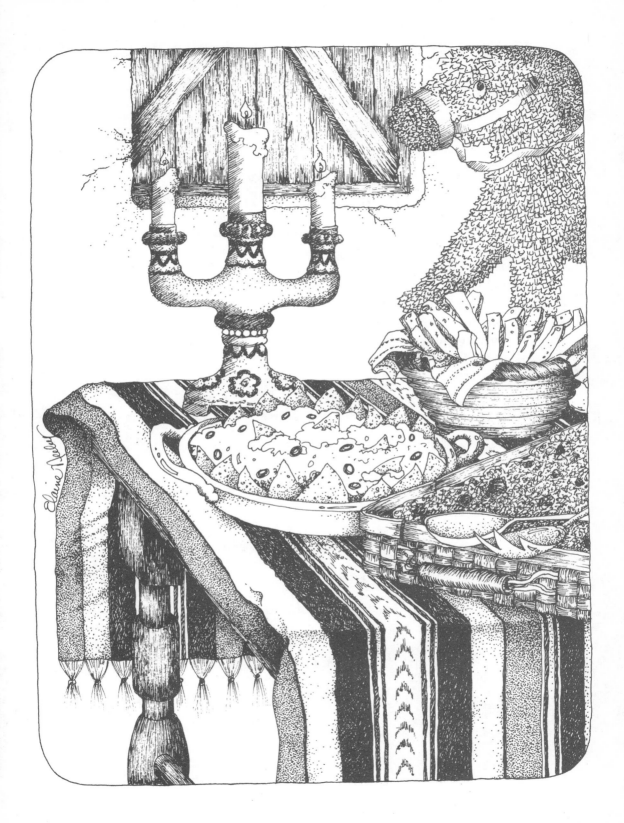

"We Must Do This More Often"

There *is* time for lunch with friends. When your turn comes, we suggest a gazebo setting with crisp white linens, flowery china, and fresh blossoms. The Layered Chicken Salad and Angel Chocolate Pie are mouth-watering specialties.

The mood of the lazy, summer day has cast its spell on your guests. "We must do this more often" are their departing words.

Ladies Luncheon

Cream of Cucumber Soup 77

Chicken-Cranberry Layered Salad 96

Asparagus Sandwiches or Tea Sandwiches 55, 56

Party Muffins 124

Angel Chocolate Pie 236

Iced Tea and Coffee

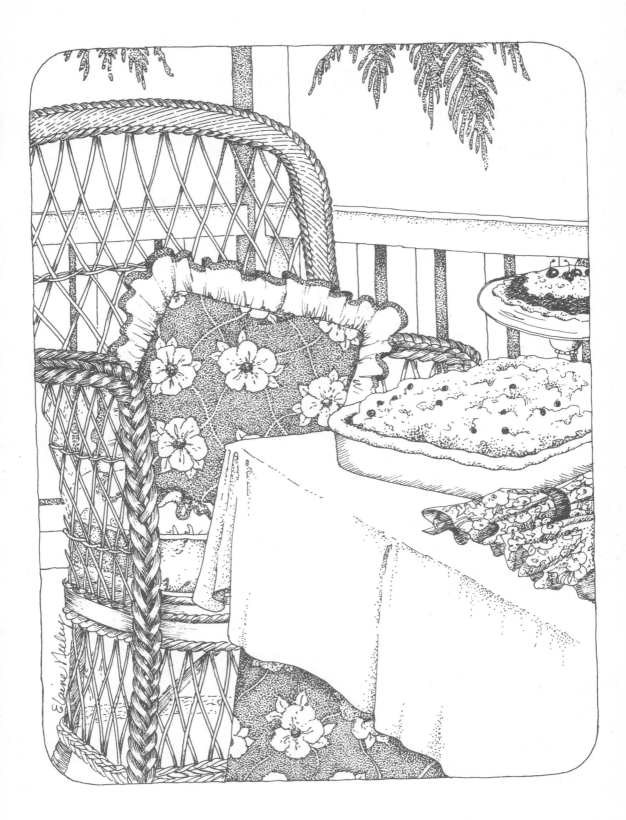

Supper of Champions

The leader board has just announced your favorite golfer as winner of the Federal Express St. Jude Classic, one of our city's outstanding entertaining opportunities. The tree-shaded porch overlooking the golf course is an inviting oasis. The wrought iron with its cool print cushions sets the mood for your hot and hungry guests. Your Porch Party with its bountiful buffet will more than satisfy.

Porch Party at the Tournament Players Club

Favorite Cocktails

Tennis Tea 74

Cheese Ring with Chutney 45

Grilled Catfish with Dijon Mustard 165

Baked Chicken Nuggets with Sweet and Sour Sauce 46, 66

Barbeque Bologna with Spicy, Spicy Mustard 36, 193

Sour Dough Bread 138

Pickled Shrimp 54

Fresh Vegetable Squares 58

Lemon Dessert Squares 283

English Toffee Squares 282

Presidential Brownies 277

Banana Ice Cream 285

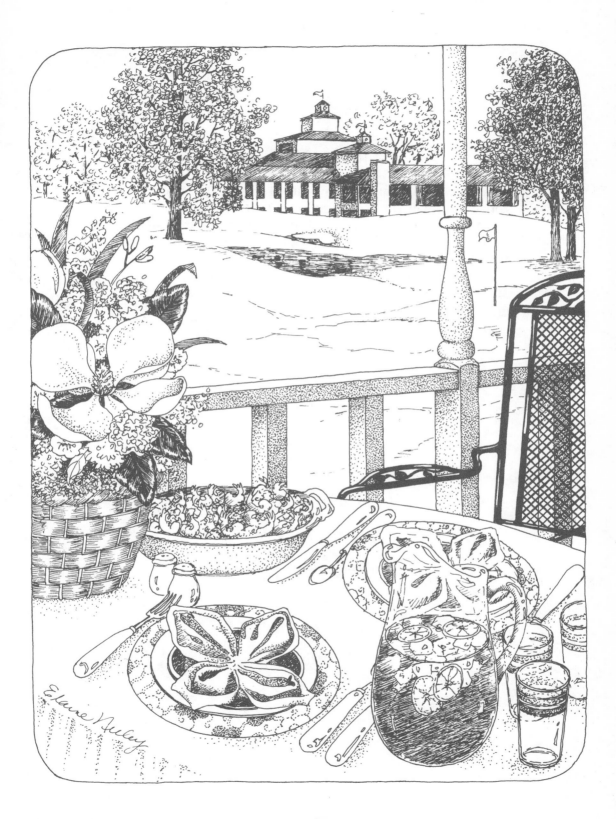

The Final Curtain

After an evening at the majestic Orpheum theatre, we continue the critique of the play over a light supper. The fun begins with Champagne Punch Cocktails and ends with a Blue Tail Fly. The very mention of that dessert conjures up memories of the Beale Street-Orpheum Theatre area. It is easy to see how Memphis' own music makers, W. C. Handy and Elvis Presley, drew their inspiration from the sights and sounds of renowned Beale Street.

After Theatre Party

Champagne Punch Cocktails 69

Party Pecans 59

Elegant Pâté with Crackers 45

Seafood Bisque 81

Green Bean Finger Sandwiches 55

Fruits in Season

Lacy Cookies 272

Blue Tail Fly 69

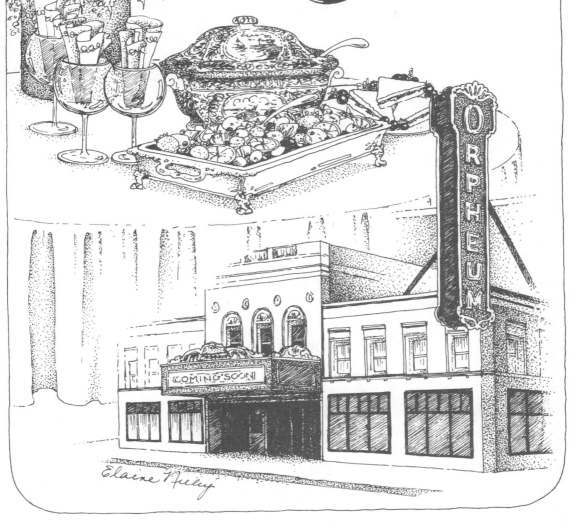

Beale St.

ORPHEUM

COMING SOON

Elaine Neely

A Feast for Football

The Delta may begin in the lobby of the Peabody Hotel, but the football season for the Mid-South begins in the parking lot of the Liberty Bowl Memorial Stadium with lively tailgate parties. When the teams take the field, whether it's the Tigers of Memphis State, the U. T. Volunteers, the Rebels of Ole Miss or the Arkansas Razorbacks, all friendships are laid aside. It's every man for himself. Appetites are hearty in the crisp fall air, so pack plenty. Bright paper plates and cups along with the largest napkins you can find are the order of the day. Don't forget a crock of wild flowers for the center of your "table".

Tailgate Party

Plantation Cheese Ball 43

Assorted Fresh Fruit Tray

Easy Shrimp Dip 63

Southern Fried Chicken 186

Baked Brisket on Rye Bread 147, 141

Calico Vegetable Salad 105

Bumpy Brownies 273

Applesauce Spice Squares 279

Sugar Cookies 271

Tailgate Beer

Chilled Wine

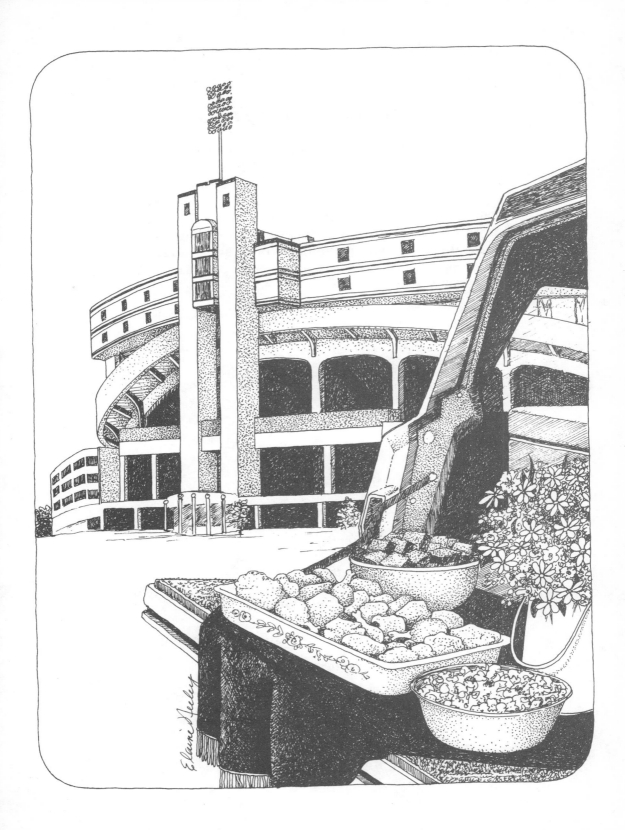

Autumn in the Fields

The bittersweet is heavy with orange clusters, and there is a little chill in the air as the riders head for home. Because so many of the dental community find themselves in the fields for any hunting season, the Hunt Brunch is something most of us have done. We suggest hunt china for this occasion. If you are lucky enough to have a stuffed pheasant, use it with persimmon, bittersweet and brass candlesticks as the table appointments. Buffet service is very traditional.

Hunt Brunch

Grilled Dove Breasts 39

Brunswick Stew 80

Garlic Cheese Grits 196

Baked Apricots or Squash Apple Bake 225, 221

Buttermilk Biscuits 119

Plum Muffins 125

Corn Light Bread 121

Coconut Pound Cake 255

Raspberry Trifle 299

Uncle Henry's Milk Punch 71

Bloody Marys

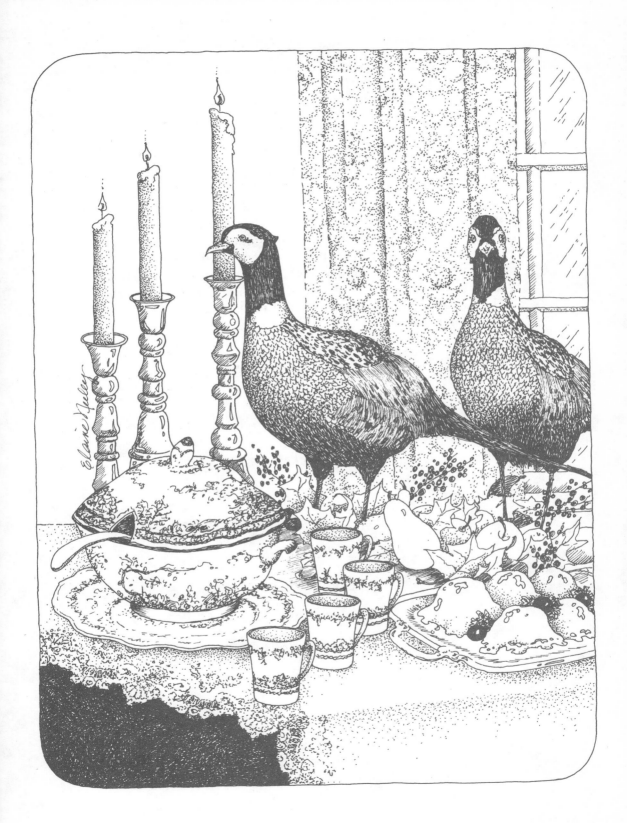

Seven o'Clock, Our Place

Because friends are so very special, pull out all of the stops. Whether you use your finest china or your latest pottery acquisition, this is a winning menu. The extra touch of seasonal flowers, fruits, or leaves will make your guests feel truly welcome. Good conversation is sure to continue with the delicious after dinner coffee and dessert. The ambiance of the evening will linger long after the guests have departed.

Dinner for Friends at Home

Oysters Rockefeller 53

Charlemagne Salad 90

Pork Tenderloin with Orange Wine Sauce 161, 195

Rice with Pine Nuts 218

Fresh Cranberry Sauce 226

Jane's Pea Casserole 214

Anybody's Rolls 132

Sherry Pie 244

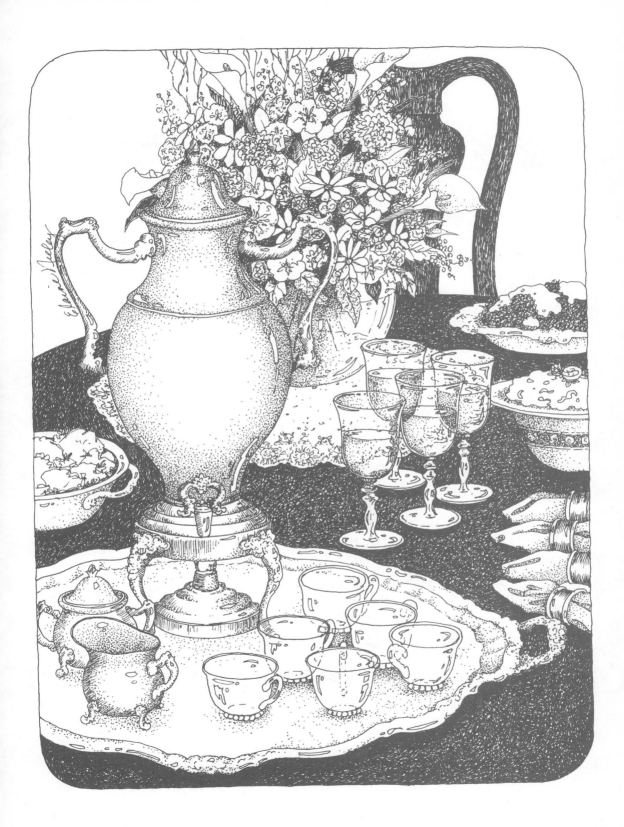

Cinnamon, Cloves, and Cousins

The big day is here. The minute you open the door, you are
carried away by the cinnamon, cloves, and sage aroma coming
from the kitchen. Family and friends wait impatiently while the
finishing touches are put to the groaning board. This is one time
when all diets are forgotten, and the entertainment is the meal
which seems to go on all day. We have gathered together our
most favorite southern dishes for this day of days. The traditional collection of recipes could also be the star attraction at
Thanksgiving time.

Holiday Dinner

Turkey and Dressing 188, 228

Giblet Gravy 193

Country Ham 158

Oyster Casserole 228

Elegant Green Bean Casserole 206

Holiday Sweet Potatoes 217

Ann's Cranberry Salad or Ambrosia Congealed Salad 89,96

Sally Lunn Bread 134

Fresh Apple Cake 245

Colonial Pecan Pie 240

Lemon Nut Cake 257

Mom's Boiled Custard 293

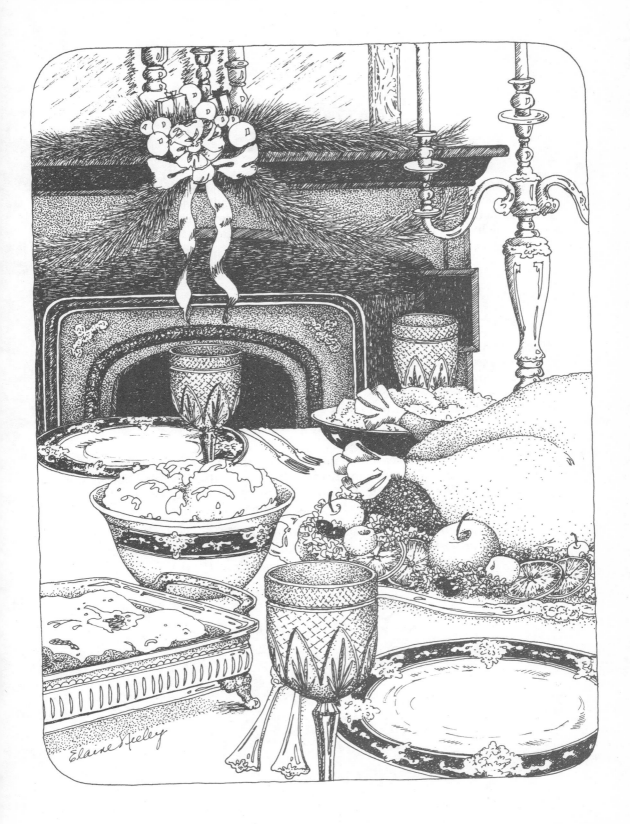

Elaine Heeley

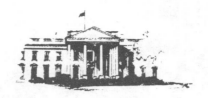

It gives us great pleasure to begin *Impressions* with this special recipe from Barbara Bush, our First Lady. She is a great inspiration to all volunteers who work to improve the quality of the lives of our citizens. We share her love of family and country.

Mexican Mound — a great Bush favorite!

A - Package of corn chips
B - 2 pounds ground meat
C - Taco seasoning mix
D - 1 cup grated yellow cheese
E - 1 or 2 small chopped onions (not minced)

F - 10 chopped ripe black olives
G - 1 chopped tomato
H - 1 cup sour cream
I - Lettuce (1 cup, shredded)
J - 1 medium can of frozen avocado dip

Follow instructions on Taco seasoning mix for browning meat. I serve this meal in my kitchen — a big pot of meat simmering on the stove, a wooden salad bowl of corn chips, and seven bowls (D through J) of the remaining ingredients around the table. Start with a mound of corn chips, a spoon of piping hot meat, cheese, etc.

Easy to make — loved by all who love Mexican food.
Ingredients easy to keep in the house. Children or guests
can all help with chopping or grating. It's fun!!

Barbara Bush

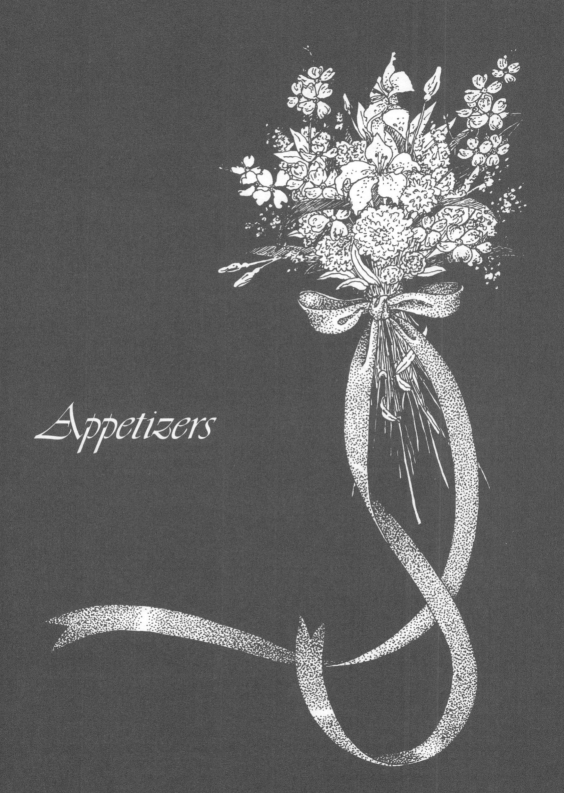

Appetizers

Antipasto

1 pint jar Giardiniera (pickled vegetables), well drained
1 (12-ounce) jar artichoke hearts in oil, undrained
1 (8-ounce) jar whole button mushrooms, drained
2 (8-ounce) cans tomato sauce
1 (7½-ounce) can tuna packed in water, drained
4 tablespoons white wine vinegar
1 (8-ounce) can pitted ripe olives, drained and halved

- Combine all ingredients, mixing well. Place in covered dish; refrigerate at least 24 hours. Keeps indefinitely in refrigerator.

- Serve with small slices of pumpernickel or rye bread.

This is a great "quickie" to precede an Italian or Spanish entrée.

Mrs. Phillip Sherman, Jr. (Sandy)

Baked Artichoke Hors d'Oeuvres

1 bunch green onions, chopped
1 garlic clove, crushed
2 (6-ounce) jars marinated artichoke hearts, drained and chopped, liquid reserved
4 eggs
12 soda crackers, crushed
8 ounces sharp cheddar cheese, shredded
2 tablespoons parsley, chopped
Salt and pepper to taste

- Preheat oven to 350 degrees.

- Sauté onions and garlic in small amount oil from artichokes.

- Beat eggs; add onion, garlic, crackers, cheese, parsley, and seasonings while beating. Fold in artichokes.

- Pour into greased 8-inch square baking dish. Bake 35 to 40 minutes. Cool and cut into squares. Serve warm. Serves 8 to 10.

- May be frozen in same pan, but always serve warm.

Mrs. James W. Clark (Carolyn)

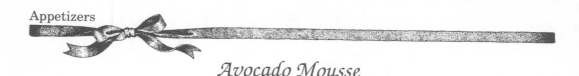

Avocado Mousse

1 (3-ounce) package lime gelatin
1 cup boiling water
2 cups mashed avocado
1 small onion, grated

½ cup mayonnaise
Juice of 1 lemon
½ teaspoon salt
¾ cup sour cream

- Dissolve gelatin in water, cool until syrupy.

- Combine avocado with onion, mayonnaise, lemon juice, and salt.

- Stir sour cream into avocado mixture. Add cooled gelatin.

- Pour into 6-cup oiled ring mold. Refrigerate until firm. Serves 6 to 8.

Mrs. Charles E. Smith (Madge)

Barbeque Bologna

1 whole bologna
2 (12-ounce) cans beer
½ cup Blue Plate barbecue sauce

1½ cups Wicker's barbecue sauce
Water

- Remove plastic wrap from bologna.

- Fill drip pan in smoker with mixture of beer, Blue Plate barbecue sauce, and Wicker's barbecue sauce, and enough water to make pan half full.

- Place bologna on rack in heated smoker and follow directions for your individual smoker.

- Smoke 4 to 5 hours turning about three times, and adding more liquid as needed to drip pan. (Liquid meaning beer, barbecue sauce, and water.)

- Serve hot off smoker with sweet hot mustard or kosher mustard on crackers as an appetizer or make sandwiches using barbecue sauce and slaw.

Mrs. J. Garland Cherry, Jr. (Carol)

Cucumber Cream Cheese Spread

1 medium cucumber, seeded and
  grated
1 small onion, grated
2 (3-ounce) packages cream cheese

Pickapeppa sauce to taste
Garlic powder to taste
Salt to taste
Mayonnaise

- Press all juice from cucumber and onion. Discard juices.

- Combine cucumber and onion with softened cream cheese and mash with fork. Add Pickapeppa, garlic, salt, and mix well.

- Mayonnaise may be added if spreading consistency needs to be adjusted. Use as dip for potato chips or spread for crackers. Serves 4 to 6.

Mrs. John Mallett Barron (Doy)

Cucumber Mousse

1 cup shredded, unpeeled cucumber
2 tablespoons grated onion
1 (3-ounce) package lime gelatin
¾ cup boiling water
1 cup small curd cottage cheese,
  mashed

1 cup mayonnaise
⅓ cup slivered almonds
Lettuce leaf

- Combine cucumber and onion. Drain well.

- Dissolve gelatin in boiling water and chill until slightly thickened.

- Fold in rest of ingredients. Spoon into 5-cup mold and chill. Unmold and serve on lettuce leaf. Serves 10 to 12.

Mrs. Frank J. Hudson (Bettye)

*P*lan on twelve hors d'oeuvres per person when determining amounts to prepare.

Baked Brie with Cranberry Chutney

⅔ cup water
⅔ cup sugar
1½ cups fresh cranberries
4 teaspoons cider vinegar
⅓ cup dark raisins
¼ cup chopped walnuts
2 teaspoons light brown sugar

Scant ¼ teaspoon ground ginger
½ teaspoon chopped garlic
1 (2¼-pound) wheel of Brie with rind
1 loaf French bread (heated and cut into thin slices)

- Preheat oven to 350 degrees.

- In heavy 3-quart saucepan, combine water and sugar. Stir to dissolve sugar; bring to boil. Add cranberries, vinegar, raisins, walnuts, brown sugar, ginger, and garlic. Boil very slowly, stirring occasionally until thick (5 minutes or longer). Remove from heat, allow to cool. Cover and refrigerate.

- Place Brie in center of rimless baking sheet lined with foil. Spread cranberry chutney over top of cheese. Fold foil loosely over cheese making a tent.

- Bake until heated thoroughly, 7 to 10 minutes. Remove from oven; lift foil and cheese to serving plate. Trim away foil and arrange greenery around cheese if desired. Serve with French bread. Serves 10 to 12.

This is especially pretty at Christmas time!

Mrs. Phillip Sherman, Jr. (Sandy)

Chicago Artichokes

1 (5¼-ounce) box Melba toast rounds
1 (13¾-ounce) can artichoke hearts, quartered and drained
⅔ cup Hellmann's mayonnaise

½ cup grated Parmesan cheese
1 tablespoon Worcestershire sauce
1 tablespoon dry sherry
¼ teaspoon onion salt
Paprika

- Preheat oven to 450 degrees.

- Cover cookie sheet with foil and place Melba rounds on cookie sheet. Put ¼ artichoke heart on each round.

- Mix mayonnaise, Parmesan cheese, Worcestershire, sherry, and onion salt together. Top each artichoke heart with 1 teaspoon of sauce. Bake 5 minutes and sprinkle with paprika. Makes 36.

Mrs. Richard L. Dixon (Ellen)
Mrs. Charles E. Harbison (Betty)

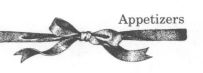

Croustades

Loaf thin white sandwich bread
Melted butter

Chili
Parmesan cheese

- Preheat oven to 400 degrees.

- Cut bread into 3-inch rounds. Lightly butter muffin or 2x1¼-inch tart tins.

- Using fingers, press bread into tins. Bake 5 minutes. Remove, turn out and cool.

- Fill croustades with chili of your choice and sprinkle with Parmesan cheese. Place on baking sheet and broil until cheese is golden. Serve warm.

- It is important to use very fresh bread! Croustades may be filled with other foods such as chicken a la king or chicken salad.

Mrs. J. Garland Cherry, Jr. (Carol)

Date and Cheese Rolls

4 ounces sharp cheddar cheese,
shredded
1 cup margarine, softened
3 cups flour, sifted

½ teaspoon salt
1 (8-ounce) package whole pitted
dates, halved
Pecans

- Preheat oven to 425 degrees.

- Cream cheese and margarine. Add flour and salt. Mix well.

- Take ½ teaspoon mixture, roll in ball and flatten. Place ½ date in middle and wrap mixture around date. Put pecan piece on top.

- Bake 10 to 15 minutes on ungreased baking sheet. Check after 10 minutes. Do not allow pecans to get too brown. Yields 84.

Mrs. Stansill Covington, III (Wrene)

Grilled Dove Breasts

24 dove breasts
12 bacon slices
1 cup Bull's Eye Barbecue sauce

1 cup Wicker's Barbecue
Marinating and Basting Sauce
2 cups Worcestershire sauce

- Wrap dove breast in one half bacon slice and secure with toothpick. Marinate two hours in sauces to cover. Grill over red hot charcoal approximately 15 minutes on each side, continually basting with sauces.

Dr. Kenneth M. Caldwell

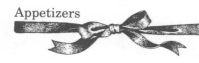

Horseradish Mold

1 envelope unflavored gelatin
3 tablespoons cold water
1 (3-ounce) package lemon gelatin
1 cup boiling water
1 (5-ounce) jar prepared
  horseradish

1 cup mayonnaise
1 cup sour cream
Garnish: sliced ripe or stuffed
  olives, pimento slices, parsley

- Dissolve unflavored gelatin in cold water. Dissolve lemon gelatin in boiling water. Mix the two together and cool slightly.

- Fold in horseradish, mayonnaise, and sour cream.

- Pour into a greased 1-quart mold. Refrigerate until set.

- Unmold and garnish with sliced ripe or stuffed olives, pimento slices, and parsley.

- Serve as a cocktail spread on crackers or serve as a side dish to roast beef.

Mrs. J. Thomas Cobb (Ann)

Tiropetakia (Cheese Puffs)

1 pound feta cheese
4 egg yolks
1 egg white, stiffly beaten
2 tablespoons Parmesan or Romano
  cheese, grated

1 pound filo pastry, thawed in
  refrigerator overnight
2 cups butter, melted

- Preheat oven to 350 degrees.

- Crumble feta cheese. Add egg yolks, stiffly beaten egg white, and Parmesan cheese.

- Cut filo pastry into 2-inch strips lengthwise. Use two strips at a time. Butter one strip, place second strip on top and butter top strip.

- Take 1 teaspoon of cheese mixture and place on the end of filo strip. Start folding into shape of a triangle (from corner to corner).

- Place on unbuttered cookie sheet. Use sheet with sides to prevent leakage in oven.

- Bake until golden brown, approximately 20 to 25 minutes. Makes approximately 70 triangles.

Can be frozen before baking or baked and then frozen.

Mrs. James G. Sousoulas (Sophie)

Cheese Bacon Triangles

1 package English muffins, split
8 ounces sharp cheddar cheese,
    shredded
6 slices bacon, cooked crisp and
    crumbled

3 tablespoons minced onion
1 (2-ounce) package slivered
    almonds, toasted and chopped
⅔ cup mayonnaise
½ teaspoon Worcestershire sauce

- Preheat oven to 400 degrees.

- Combine cheese, bacon, onion, almonds, mayonnaise, and Worcestershire sauce and spread on muffins. Cut muffins in fourths and place on ungreased cookie sheet.

- Bake for about 10 minutes. Serve warm.

These may be frozen uncooked. Thaw before baking.

Mrs. Justin D. Towner (Ginny)

Cheddar Cheese Spread

⅓ cup evaporated milk
⅛ teaspoon minced garlic
2 tablespoons butter
8 ounces sharp cheddar cheese,
    shredded

1 (4-ounce) can chopped green
    chilies, undrained
Dash cayenne

- Heat milk to boiling, add garlic and butter.

- Pour over cheese and beat until smooth.

- Add chilies and cayenne.

- Chill for several hours before serving.

- Serve on sesame or cheddar cracker sticks.

Mrs. Charles B. Lansden (Ann)

My Caviar Cheese Ball

1 (8-ounce) package cream cheese, softened
Onion powder

2 ounces red or black caviar
Juice of ½ lemon

• Mold cream cheese into ball. Sprinkle with onion powder and spread with caviar.

• Spray lemon juice over all as a mist. Serves 8 to 10.

*Cream cheese may be made into any shape,
such as Christmas tree using red caviar.*

Mrs. Ralph Waldo Handy (Sharolene)

Cheddar Cheese Ball

8 ounces cheddar cheese, shredded
1 (3-ounce) package cream cheese
½ teaspoon garlic powder
½ teaspoon onion powder
¼ teaspoon salt

¼ teaspoon Worcestershire sauce
⅛ teaspoon red pepper
¾ cup chopped pecans
Chili powder

• Mix and roll in chili powder.

Mrs. Donald W. Crone (Pat)

Pimento Cheese Ball

1 (10-ounce) package shredded cheddar cheese
1 (8-ounce) package cream cheese, softened
1 (3-ounce) package cream cheese, softened

3 tablespoons chopped sweet pickle or pickle relish
3 tablespoons diced pimento, drained
3 tablespoons minced onion
1 cup chopped pecans

• Combine cheeses, pickle, pimento, and onion. Chill. Form ball and roll in pecans. Serve with assorted crackers.

Variation: Roll in snipped parsley instead of pecans.

Mrs. Michael J. Harty (Kay)

Pineapple Cheese Ball

2 (8-ounce) packages cream cheese,
   softened
1 (8-ounce) can crushed pineapple,
   well drained
¼ cup finely chopped green bell
   pepper

2 tablespoons minced onion
1 tablespoon seasoned salt
2 cups chopped pecans

- Combine cream cheese, pineapple, green bell pepper, onion, salt, and 1 cup of pecans. Chill 10 minutes.

- Form into ball and roll in other cup of pecans. Chill until ready to serve. Serves 16.

Mrs. Carl Cutting (Jo Ann)

Plantation Cheese Ball

2 (8-ounce) packages cream cheese
2 cups finely chopped pecans
½ teaspoon Worcestershire sauce
½ teaspoon salt

¼ teaspoon Tabasco
Garlic powder to taste
¼ teaspoon paprika

- Blend all ingredients except paprika. Shape into ball, wrap in plastic wrap and chill. Sprinkle with paprika when ready to serve.

Mrs. John Mallett Barron (Doy)

Cheese Wafers

8 ounces sharp cheddar cheese,
   shredded
½ cup margarine
½ cup butter
2 cups flour

2 eggs, beaten
Pecan halves
Salt
Paprika

- Preheat oven to 375 degrees.

- Mix cheese, margarine, butter, and flour. Roll thin and cut in 1¾-inch circles. Brush top with beaten egg and place pecan half on each circle.

- Bake 10 to 15 minutes. Sprinkle lightly with salt and paprika while hot. Makes 100.

Mrs. J. Roy Bourgoyne (Helen Ruth)

Mother's Cheese Wafers

½ cup margarine
1 cup flour
1 teaspoon salt
2 cups shredded sharp cheddar
cheese

¼ teaspoon red pepper
¾ cup chopped pecans

- Mix all ingredients and form into a log. Refrigerate.

- Preheat oven to 400 degrees.

- When ready to bake, cut into thin slices and place on a cookie sheet. Bake 10 minutes.

- May substitute 2 cups Rice Krispies for pecans. Makes 48.

Mrs. Charles E. Harbison (Betty)
Mrs. Sidney Friedman, Jr. (Ann)

Sesame Cheese Straws

1 (2½-ounce) jar sesame seed
8 ounces sharp cheddar cheese,
shredded
1¼ cups flour

½ cup butter or margarine,
softened
⅛ teaspoon cayenne
1 teaspoon salt

- Preheat oven to 375 degrees.

- Toast sesame seed in a heavy skillet, stirring constantly over low heat about 20 minutes or until golden brown, cool. Set aside.

- Combine remaining ingredients; work dough until mixture is well blended. Add sesame seed. Roll dough to ⅛-inch thickness. Cut into 4x½-inch strips.

- Bake on ungreased sheet for 12 to 15 minutes. Cool on wire rack. Yields 60.

These keep several weeks in airtight container.

Mrs. Carl L. Sebelius, Jr. (Judy)

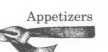

Cheese Ring with Chutney

1 pound cheddar cheese, shredded
¾ cup mayonnaise
1 cup chopped pecans
½ medium onion, finely chopped

½ teaspoon garlic salt
½ teaspoon Tabasco
1 small jar chutney
Lettuce leaves

- Combine cheese, mayonnaise, pecans, onion, garlic salt, and Tabasco. Place in small greased bundt pan or ring pan. Refrigerate 24 hours.

- Remove from pan, place on bed of lettuce and put chutney in center of ring.

Variation: Pepper jelly or strawberry preserves may be substituted for chutney.

Mrs. H. Franklin Miller (Carolyn)
Mrs. Joe L. Cannon (Nell)

Elegant Pâté

1½ pounds chicken livers
½ small onion
Water
Salt
1 cup butter or margarine, softened
⅓ cup minced onion
1 teaspoon salt

⅛ teaspoon cayenne
1 tablespoon dry mustard
¼ teaspoon ground nutmeg
⅛ teaspoon cloves
Lettuce leaves (optional)
Chopped hard-boiled eggs
  (optional)

- Cook livers and onion half in boiling salted water to cover until tender, about 15 minutes. Drain.

- Place cooked chicken livers, butter, minced onion, salt, cayenne, mustard, nutmeg, and cloves in container of electric blender or food processor. Process until smooth, turn into buttered mold. Cover and chill several hours.

- When ready to serve, turn onto lettuce leaf and garnish with chopped hard-boiled eggs. Good with assorted crackers. Makes about 2 cups.

May be made several days in advance.

Mrs. Phillip Sherman, Jr. (Sandy)

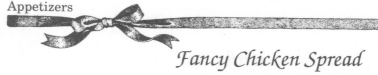

Fancy Chicken Spread

2 (8-ounce) packages cream cheese, softened
1 tablespoon A-1 bottled steak sauce
1 teaspoon curry powder
2 chicken breasts, cooked and finely chopped

¼ cup chopped celery
1 tablespoon grated onion
¼ cup minced green bell pepper
¾ cup chopped parsley
¼ cup chopped almonds

• Beat together cream cheese, steak sauce, and curry powder. Add chicken, celery, onion, green bell pepper, and 2 tablespoons of parsley.

• Shape into a log, wrap in plastic wrap and chill 4 hours or overnight. Toss together remaining parsley and almonds and use to coat log. Serve with crackers. Serves 14 to 16.

Variation: Omit curry.

Mrs. Frank J. Hudson (Bettye)

Baked Chicken Nuggets

7 to 8 whole chicken breasts, boned and skinned
2 cups fine breadcrumbs
1 cup grated Parmesan cheese
3 tablespoons sesame seed
1½ teaspoons salt

1 tablespoon plus 1 teaspoon dried whole thyme
1 tablespoon plus 1 teaspoon dried whole basil
1 cup butter or margarine, melted

• Preheat oven to 400 degrees.

• Cut chicken into 1½-inch pieces.

• Combine breadcrumbs, cheese, sesame seed, salt, and herbs. Mix well.

• Dip chicken pieces in butter and coat with breadcrumb mixture. Place on ungreased baking sheet in a single layer. Bake 20 minutes or until done.

• Serve with a sweet 'n sour sauce or Tangy Dipping Sauce (see index). Serves 14 to 16.

Mrs. James E. Sexton (Pat)

Sesame Chicken Strips

2½ to 3 pounds boneless chicken
   breasts, cut into strips
2 tablespoons butter, melted
¼ cup sesame seed, toasted

3 teaspoons salt
½ teaspoon ground black pepper
⅛ teaspoon garlic powder
½ cup flour

- Preheat oven to 400 degrees.

- Dip or brush each piece of chicken with melted butter.

- Put remaining ingredients in paper bag. Add chicken and shake well to coat each piece.

- Place chicken in 13x9x2-inch pan. Bake approximately 15 minutes, turning once to brown evenly. Serve with toothpicks. Serves 6 to 8.

Mrs. James E. Sexton (Pat)

Cocktail Meatballs

1 pound ground chuck
½ cup dry breadcrumbs
⅓ cup minced onion
¼ cup milk
1 egg
1 tablespoon snipped parsley

1 teaspoon salt
⅛ teaspoon pepper
½ teaspoon Worcestershire sauce
¼ cup cooking oil
1 (12-ounce) bottle chili sauce
1 (10-ounce) jar grape jelly

- Mix ground chuck, breadcrumbs, onion, milk, egg, and next four ingredients together. Gently shape into 1-inch balls.

- Put oil in large skillet and lightly brown meatballs. Remove from skillet and pour off drippings.

- Heat chili sauce and jelly in skillet, stirring constantly until jelly is melted. Add meatballs and stir until thoroughly coated. Simmer uncovered 30 minutes. Makes 5 dozen.

Mrs. H. Ray Manning (Rose Marie)

Sweet and Sour Meatballs

1 pound hot sausage
1 pound ground chuck
½ cup ketchup
½ cup brown sugar

¼ teaspoon ginger
½ cup wine vinegar
1 tablespoon soy sauce

- Preheat oven to 350 degrees.

- Combine sausage and ground chuck. Shape into balls and bake about 35 minutes on slotted broiler pan.

- Combine ketchup, sugar, ginger, vinegar, and soy sauce and marinate meatballs in this sauce for 24 hours.

- Reheat meatballs and sauce. Serve hot in chafing dish. Yields about 60.

Mrs. Joe Hall Morris (Adair)

Mushroom Turnovers

Filling:
3 tablespoons butter
1 onion, minced
12 ounces fresh mushrooms,
   chopped
½ teaspoon salt

Dash pepper
2 teaspoons flour
½ cup sour cream
1 teaspoon dried dill

- Melt butter; sauté onion and mushrooms. Add salt, pepper, and flour. Cook 2 minutes. Remove from heat. Add sour cream and dill. Chill.

Pastry:
1 (8-ounce) package cream cheese,
   softened
1 cup margarine, softened
⅛ teaspoon salt

2 cups flour, sifted
1 egg yolk
2 teaspoons milk

- Blend cream cheese and margarine. Add salt and flour; mix until a smooth pastry dough is formed. Chill.

- Place pastry on sheet of floured waxed paper, top with another sheet of waxed paper, and roll pastry to ¼-inch thickness.

- Cut with 3-inch biscuit cutter. Place 1½ teaspoons filling on each round of dough. Fold pastry in half and press edges firmly with fork. Combine egg yolk and milk to make a wash. Brush tops of turnovers with wash. Freeze.

- Bake frozen at 350 degrees 15 to 20 minutes. Makes 65.

Cookbook Committee

Stuffed Mushrooms

24 large whole mushrooms
3 tablespoons vegetable oil
1/3 pound ground beef
1 medium onion, finely chopped
3 slices ham, coarsely chopped
1/2 cup sherry

1/3 cup fine breadcrumbs
1 teaspoon salt
1 teaspoon pepper
1 1/2 teaspoons garlic powder
1/3 cup grated Parmesan cheese

- Preheat broiler of oven.

- Remove stems from mushrooms and chop finely. Place caps underside up on cookie sheet.

- Heat oil in large skillet over medium heat, add beef and onion; cook until lightly browned. Add chopped stems, ham, and sherry to beef mixture. Cook 5 minutes. Add breadcrumbs, salt, pepper, and garlic powder and mix well.

- Stuff mixture into mushroom caps. Sprinkle with cheese. Broil 3 to 4 inches from heat for 2 to 5 minutes. Serve hot.

Mrs. John Tillman (Joanne)

Sausage Stuffed Mushrooms

1 pound fresh mushrooms
1 pound pork sausage
1 teaspoon minced garlic
2 tablespoons chopped parsley,
   or 1 tablespoon if using dried

6 ounces sharp cheddar cheese,
   shredded

- Preheat oven to 350 degrees.

- Rinse mushrooms and pat dry. Remove stems.

- Chop stems and combine with sausage, garlic, and parsley. Cook until sausage is browned, stirring to crumble. Drain. Stir in cheese, mixing well.

- Spoon mixture into mushrooms and place in 13x9x2-inch ungreased dish. Work fast while mixture is warm or it will start hardening. Bake 20 minutes. Yields 24.

Mrs. Phillip Sherman, Jr. (Sandy)

Sausage Swirls

½ pound hot sausage
½ pound mild sausage
2 (8-ounce) cans crescent dinner
  rolls

2 tablespoons hot mustard

- Preheat oven to 325 degrees when ready to bake.

- Cook and drain sausage.

- Separate rolls into 4 rectangles. Spread rolls with mustard and sprinkle sausage over mustard. Roll dough up jelly roll fashion.

- Chill overnight. Slice each section into 10 slices. Bake 10 to 15 minutes on lightly greased cookie sheet. Serve warm. Makes 40 swirls.

Mrs. Phillip Sherman, Sr. (Barbara)

Dolmathakia (Stuffed Grapevine Leaves)

1 (16-ounce) jar grapevine leaves
Warm water
2 cups long grain rice
1 cup olive oil (reserve
  3 tablespoons)
2 cups water
1 bunch green onions or 2 large
  onions, finely chopped

2 teaspoons salt
¼ teaspoon pepper
2 tablespoons chopped parsley
2 tablespoons chopped dill,
  preferably fresh
Juice of 3 lemons, divided

- Place grapevine leaves in bowl of warm water for 15 minutes before using. Set aside.

- Combine rice, oil, water, onions, salt, pepper, parsley, dill, and juice of 2 lemons in saucepan. Place over high heat, stirring constantly, until mixture comes to a boil. Lower heat and simmer until most of liquid is absorbed. Remove from heat and drain in colander.

- Place 1 teaspoon of rice mixture in center of grapevine leaf, fold sides in, and loosely roll up. Arrange in layers in Dutch oven adding reserved 3 tablespoons olive oil, juice of 1 lemon, and enough water to cover rolls. Place heavy plate over rolls.

- Cover saucepan and cook slowly until most of liquid is absorbed and rice is tender. Additional water may be added if necessary. Makes 36. These can be made ahead and kept in refrigerator or freezer. Do not freeze in plastic wrap.

*Serve hot or cold as delicious appetizer
or luncheon dish with lamb or chicken.*

Mrs. James G. Sousoulas (Sophie)

Shrimp Tomato Mold

2 (10¾-ounce) cans undiluted
tomato soup
2 (3-ounce) packages cream cheese
3 packages unflavored gelatin
½ cup wine vinegar
¼ cup lemon juice
½ cup ketchup
1½ pounds small shrimp, cooked,
shelled, and halved

2 cups (combined) finely chopped
green bell pepper, onion, and
celery
1 cup mayonnaise
Dash Tabasco
Dash Worcestershire sauce

- Heat soup and cream cheese until cheese is melted. Add gelatin. Let cool. Add remaining ingredients.

- Pour ingredients in lightly oiled 3-quart mold to congeal. Unmold; serve with your favorite crackers.

Mrs. Frank J. Hudson (Bettye)
Mrs. Jack C. Shannon (Judy)

Southern Crab Dip

1¼ cups mayonnaise
⅔ cup sour cream
2¼ tablespoons French dressing
1¼ teaspoons horseradish
2½ teaspoons Worcestershire sauce

¼ teaspoon salt
⅛ teaspoon pepper
1 (16-ounce) package shredded
cheddar cheese
2½ pounds crabmeat

- Blend together mayonnaise and sour cream. Add French dressing, horseradish, Worcestershire, salt, and pepper.

- Mix in cheese and crabmeat. Stir lightly and refrigerate.

This should be made one day in advance.

Mrs. Joe L. Cannon (Nell)

Hollow out a red cabbage and use it for a bowl for your favorite dip.

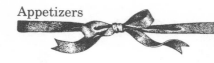

Crab Pâté

1 envelope unflavored gelatin
3 tablespoons cold water
1 (10¾-ounce) can cream of celery
   soup
¾ cup mayonnaise
1 (8-ounce) package cream cheese,
   softened
1 cup or 1 (6-ounce) can crabmeat,
   rinsed and drained

½ small onion, minced
1 cup minced celery
Salad greens
Shrimp
Sliced mushrooms
Ripe olives
Crackers

- Soften gelatin in cold water.

- Heat soup and stir in gelatin until dissolved. Add mayonnaise and cream cheese; blend well.

- Stir in crabmeat, onion, and celery.

- Spray 1-quart mold with vegetable spray. Pour in pâté and chill overnight. Unmold on a bed of salad greens and garnish with shrimp, sliced mushrooms, and ripe olives. Serve with crackers. Yields 4 cups.

Mrs. John Hembree (Mary Ellen)

Crab Rolls

¾ cup butter
1 pound Velveeta cheese, cubed
2 (6-ounce) cans crabmeat, flaked
1 (24-ounce) loaf very fresh white
   sandwich bread, crust removed

¾ cup butter, melted
1 ounce sesame seed

- Melt ¾ cup butter and cheese in double boiler or microwave. Add crab.

- Using rolling pin, flatten each slice of bread until paper thin. Spread crab mixture on bread and roll up like jelly roll.

- Roll each sandwich in melted butter and then in sesame seed.

- Freeze on cookie sheet. Before cooking, thaw for 15 minutes. Cut into halves or thirds and broil until lightly browned, turning once. Serve immediately.

Mrs. Richard M. Thompson (Debby)

Crabmeat Mornay

½ cup margarine
5 to 6 green onions, chopped
½ cup parsley, finely chopped
2 tablespoons flour
2 cups half-and-half

8 ounces Swiss cheese, shredded
¼ cup dry sherry
Salt and pepper to taste
1 pound crabmeat

• Melt margarine. Sauté onions and parsley. Blend in flour and cream. Add cheese and stir until melted.

• Add sherry and seasonings and gently fold in crabmeat. Serves 6 to 8.

Mrs. L. C. Templeton (Virginia)

Oysters Rockefeller

4 dozen oysters

1 box of rock salt

• Shuck oysters, removing each individual oyster and wash well.

• Pat oysters dry with paper towel. Place dry oysters back in shell and put on a bed of rock salt on flat pan. Broil in oven until edges curl, approximately 6 to 8 minutes.

• Remove oysters and drain liquid from shell.

Sauce:
2 (10-ounce) packages frozen
  spinach, cooked and drained
1 bunch green onions, chopped
1 bunch parsley, minced
1 stalk celery, chopped
1 cup butter, melted
2 cups breadcrumbs
4 tablespoons Worcestershire sauce

1 teaspoon anise seed
2 to 4 tablespoons Perino liqueur
  to taste
Salt and pepper to taste
Dash cayenne
Parmesan cheese
Paprika

• Preheat oven to 400 degrees.

• Grind all greens in blender or food processor. Add melted butter, breadcrumbs, Worcestershire, anise seed, Perino, salt, pepper, and cayenne.

• Add sauce to cover oysters. Top with Parmesan cheese and paprika. Bake 10 minutes, or until cheese browns.

Dr. Robert Ducklo

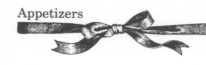

Pickled Shrimp

1 large onion, sliced
2 lemons, sliced
2 pounds shrimp, cooked, shelled,
  and deveined
1 bay leaf
1 cup oil
½ cup vinegar

1 (10¾-ounce) can tomato soup
½ teaspoon garlic salt
½ teaspoon paprika
½ teaspoon red pepper
½ teaspoon dry mustard
½ teaspoon Worcestershire sauce

- Layer onion, lemons, shrimp, and bay leaf in 13x9x2-inch pyrex dish.

- Blend remaining ingredients and pour over shrimp.

- Cover bowl and marinate 24 to 48 hours. Serves 4 to 6.

Mrs. Carl L. Sebelius, Jr. (Judy)

Snow Peas with Boursin

50 to 60 tender snow peas
1 (4-ounce) package Boursin cheese

Small mint leaves

- Remove stem end from peas, string and blanch in a large pot of rapidly boiling water for 30 seconds. Plunge them immediately into cool water to stop the cooking and preserve their green color.

- With a small sharp knife, slit open the straight seam of each pea and pipe the softened cheese into each.

- Garnish each pod with a small mint leaf.

Cookbook Committee

Use cottage cheese in dips rather than sour cream to save calories.

Asparagus Sandwiches

1 (10½-ounce) can asparagus tips, drained
1 (8-ounce) package cream cheese, softened
2 hard-boiled eggs, finely chopped
2 tablespoons lemon juice
1 teaspoon seasoned salt
½ cup (or more) margarine, melted
1 loaf sandwich bread, crust removed
Parmesan cheese

- Combine asparagus, cream cheese, eggs, lemon juice, and salt. Mix until smooth.

- Brush margarine on inside of bread. Spread with asparagus mixture and top with bread. Brush outside of sandwiches with melted margarine. Sprinkle cheese on outside and broil on both sides.

- May be baked at 400 degrees 10 to 15 minutes.

- Sandwiches may be frozen. Omit Parmesan cheese until thawed and ready to cook. Makes 14 sandwiches.

A luncheon favorite!

Mrs. J. Roy Bourgoyne (Helen Ruth)

Green Bean Finger Sandwiches

2 (16-ounce) cans whole blue lake green beans, drained
2 (8-ounce) bottles Italian salad dressing
1 loaf sandwich bread
Mayonnaise
Spicy brown mustard

- Marinate green beans in Italian dressing overnight.

- Trim crust from bread. Press each slice with rolling pin to flatten.

- Mix mayonnaise and mustard in equal parts and spread on one side of bread. Place 2 green beans on edge of bread and roll. Press together lightly. Cut into bite size pieces. Serves 30.

You must try this. It's great for a tea.

Mrs. Richard C. Harris (Beverly)

Mini Reuben Sandwiches

2 loaves party rye bread
1 cup butter, softened
1½ cups Thousand Island dressing
2 cups sauerkraut, rinsed and
   drained

1 pound sliced corned beef, cut into
   small squares
1 pound sliced Swiss cheese, cut
   into small squares

- Butter a slice of bread, spread with dressing, top with kraut, corned beef, cheese and top with another slice of buttered bread which has been spread with dressing. Repeat with remaining ingredients.

- Butter electric skillet and cook sandwiches on medium until brown; turn and brown other side. Serve with slice of dill pickle. Yields 48.

Mrs. John Hembree (Mary Ellen)

Tea Sandwiches

Green bell pepper
Pecans

Hellmann's mayonnaise
Roman Meal bread

- Finely chop equal portions of green bell pepper and pecans. Add enough mayonnaise to moisten so that mixture is of spreading consistency.

- Cut crust from slices of bread and spread mixture on half the slices and top with remaining slices. Cut sandwiches into thirds.

Mrs. James F. Bennett, Jr. (Ann)
Mrs. L. C. Templeton (Virginia)

Prepare sandwiches the day before and cover with wax paper and damp kitchen towel to retain freshness.

Quiche Individual

2 (3-ounce) packages cream cheese
1 cup butter
2 cups flour
3 eggs, beaten
2 cups half-and-half

1 teaspoon salt
1 teaspoon Worcestershire sauce
½ teaspoon dry mustard
1 (3¼-ounce) bottle bacon bits
6 ounces Swiss cheese, shredded

- Preheat oven to 350 degrees.

- Cream cheese, butter, and flour. Pinch off small pieces of dough and press in bottom and up sides of smallest muffin pans.

- Mix eggs with half-and-half and seasonings.

- Sprinkle bacon bits on bottom of muffin tart, then a good pinch of cheese. Pour egg mixture over all.

- Bake 30 minutes or until nicely brown on top. Serve warm. Yields 48 muffins.

Mrs. A. G. Baxter (Frances)

Swiss Bacon Lorraine

1 (8-ounce) package refrigerated
  crescent rolls
4 slices Swiss cheese
3 eggs, slightly beaten
¾ cup milk

1 tablespoon minced onion
4 slices bacon, cooked crisp and
  crumbled
1 tablespoon parsley flakes

- Preheat oven to 425 degrees.

- Press crescent rolls onto bottom and 1-inch up sides of a greased 8-inch square baking dish. Place cheese over dough.

- Combine eggs, milk, and onion. Pour over cheese. Sprinkle bacon and parsley on top of all ingredients. Bake 15 to 18 minutes. Cool, cut into squares. Serves 10.

Mrs. Tony Hughey (Carol)

Spinach Appetizers

2 eggs, beaten
1 (10-ounce) package frozen
chopped spinach, drained
¼ cup melted butter
1 pound Monterey Jack cheese,
shredded

1 cup milk
¾ cup flour
1 teaspoon salt
1 teaspoon baking powder

- Preheat oven to 350 degrees.

- Combine all ingredients and pour into buttered 13x9x2-inch pan.

- Bake 40 to 45 minutes. Cool a few minutes. Cut in small squares. Serve hot or cold. Makes 30 to 40 squares.

Mrs. Phillip Sherman, Jr. (Sandy)

Fresh Vegetable Squares

2 packages crescent rolls
1 (1-ounce) package dry ranch
dressing mix
2 (8-ounce) containers softened
cream cheese
1 cup mayonnaise

1 cup shredded cheddar cheese
1 cup chopped broccoli
1 cup chopped cauliflower
⅓ cup chopped onion
½ cup chopped celery
½ cup chopped carrots

- Preheat oven to 375 degrees.

- Unroll each package of crescent rolls onto a 15x10-inch pan. Use your fingers and rolling pin to stretch dough to cover the pan. Pinch together the seams. Bake 5 to 7 minutes.

- Mix ranch dressing, cream cheese, and mayonnaise. Stir until mixture is blended and smooth. Spread over pastry.

- Top with cheese and chopped vegetables. Lightly press down and refrigerate. When ready to serve cut into 2x2-inch squares. Serves 35.

Mrs. Joe Hall Morris (Adair)

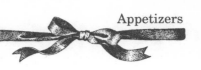

Party Pecans

1 pound pecan halves
¼ cup margarine, melted

Salt

- Preheat oven to 325 degrees.

- Place pecan halves on foil lined 15x10x1-inch jelly-roll pan. Brush half of melted margarine on pecans. Salt pecans generously.

- Bake 10 minutes and remove from oven. Turn pecans, brush on remaining margarine, and salt generously. Return to oven and bake 5 minutes. Remove from oven, turn, and bake 3 to 4 minutes, or until toasted golden brown.

- Turn onto waxed paper, salt generously, and cool.

Store in tin and serve within 2 or 3 days
Mrs. David R. Libby (Donna)

Seasoned Oyster Crackers

1 (11-ounce) box oyster crackers
1 (1-ounce) package dry ranch dressing mix

½ cup corn oil
1½ teaspoons dill weed

- Mix all ingredients. Let stand 5 or 10 minutes. Mix again.

Mrs. Lee. E. Wilson (Carol)

Fresh Vegetable Mousse

1 envelope unflavored gelatin
¼ cup cold water
¼ cup boiling water
2 cups mayonnaise
1 teaspoon salt
1 cucumber, peeled, minced, and well drained

2 tomatoes, minced and well drained
1 cup minced celery
1 small onion, minced
1 green bell pepper, minced

- In large bowl, dissolve gelatin in cold water, then add boiling water. Cool to room temperature.

- Fold mayonnaise and salt in gelatin mixture. Add vegetables and mix. Pour in 1½-quart mold and refrigerate until firm. Serve with crackers.

Mrs. Dwight A. Morris (Cathy)

Artichoke Dip

1 (14-ounce) can artichokes,
drained and chopped
½ cup chopped onion
1 cup mayonnaise

1 cup freshly grated Parmesan
cheese
1 (4-ounce) can sliced mushrooms,
drained

- Preheat oven to 350 degrees.

- Mix artichokes, onion, mayonnaise, and cheese together. Fold in sliced mushrooms.

- Place in ungreased 8-inch square baking dish, and bake uncovered 25 minutes. Serve warm with chips or crackers. Serves 8 to 10.

*This dip is good uncooked too. For variation add
1 (4-ounce) can green chilies, chopped and drained.*

*Mrs. H. Ray Manning (Rose Marie)
Mrs. Jack E. Wells (Genie)*

Broccoli Dip

1 medium onion, chopped
¼ cup margarine
2 (10-ounce) packages frozen
chopped broccoli, cooked and
drained

1 (10¾-ounce) can cream of
mushroom soup
1 (4-ounce) can chopped
mushrooms, drained
1 (6-ounce) roll garlic cheese

- Sauté onion in margarine until soft. Add broccoli, soup, mushrooms, and cheese and stir until cheese is melted.

- Serve in chafing dish with crackers or corn chips. Serves 12.

Variation: Add ½ cup chopped celery sautéed in margarine. Substitute 1 (6-ounce) roll jalapeño pepper cheese for garlic cheese.

May also be used as a vegetable casserole.

*Mrs. James D. Higgason (Nancy)
Mrs. Fernando C. Heros (Gayle)*

Hot Bean Dip

1 (16-ounce) can refried beans
1 cup canned tomatoes, chopped
and drained
1 (4-ounce) can chopped green
chilies, undrained

8 ounces Monterey Jack or sharp
cheddar cheese, shredded
¼ teaspoon onion powder
¼ teaspoon salt
¼ teaspoon garlic powder

• Combine all ingredients. Heat until cheese is melted. If too thick, add some tomato juice. Serve hot with corn chips. Yields 5 cups.

Mrs. Frank J. Hudson (Bettye)

Dill Dip

⅔ cup mayonnaise
⅔ cup sour cream
1 tablespoon thinly sliced green
onion

1 tablespoon dried parsley
1 teaspoon dried dill weed
1 teaspoon seasoned salt

• Mix all ingredients and chill.

Mrs. David R. Libby (Donna)

Dip for a Crowd

2 chicken breast halves, cooked and
chopped
1 (10¾-ounce) can cream of
mushroom soup
1 (3-ounce) can mushroom pieces,
undrained

1 (2-ounce) package slivered
almonds
1 (8-ounce) package cream cheese
1 teaspoon Worcestershire sauce
⅛ teaspoon garlic salt

• Mix all ingredients together and heat thoroughly.

• Serve warm with large corn chips. Approximately 35 servings.

May substitute 1 (6¾-ounce) can boneless chicken, crab or tuna.

Mrs. J. Roy Bourgoyne (Helen Ruth)

Nina's Clam Dip

3 (8-ounce) packages cream cheese
3 (6½-ounce) cans minced clams, undrained
1 (4-ounce) can mushrooms, sliced and drained
½ cup chopped chives or green onions

1 garlic clove, minced
⅛ teaspoon salt
1 tablespoon soy sauce
1 tablespoon Worcestershire sauce

• Melt cheese in double boiler. Add remaining ingredients and mix well.

• Serve warm in chafing dish or fondue pot with crackers. Yields 4 to 6 cups.

Mrs. Richard J. Reynolds (Anne)

Hot Crab Dip

2 (8-ounce) packages cream cheese
1 (8-ounce) carton sour cream
2 (6-ounce) cans crabmeat, flaked
1 teaspoon prepared horseradish

2 tablespoons grated onion, drained
2 tablespoons white wine
1 (2-ounce) package slivered almonds, toasted

• Preheat oven to 300 degrees.

• Melt cream cheese in double boiler or microwave. Add sour cream, crab, horseradish, onion, and wine. Stir until mixed well.

• Place in 1½-quart round buttered casserole. Bake uncovered 15 minutes. Increase oven temperature to 350 degrees for additional 15 minutes or until hot and bubbly.

• Place in chafing dish and sprinkle almonds on top. Serve with assorted crackers.

Mrs. N. Edward Tillman (Ann)

Cream cheese will slice and spread better if it is at room temperature.

Easy Shrimp Dip

1 (4½-ounce) can tiny shrimp
2 teaspoons lemon juice
1 cup sour cream

1 (8-ounce) package cream cheese
1 (0.7-ounce) package Good Seasons
   Italian dressing mix

- Rinse and drain shrimp. Combine remaining ingredients and mix until smooth. Add shrimp. Refrigerate at least 3 hours before serving.

- Serve with assorted crackers or chips. Makes 2 cups.

Miss Traci Sherman

Fruit Dip

1 (8-ounce) carton strawberry
   yogurt
1 (8-ounce) carton whipped topping

1 (3-ounce) package cream cheese,
   softened (optional)

- Combine all ingredients. Makes 3 to 4 cups.

Sliced apples are especially good with this dip.
Hint: Soak apples in pineapple juice to prevent darkening.

Mrs. Lesley H. Binkley, Jr. (Nancy)

Holiday Salmon Dip

2 (6½-ounce) cans pink salmon,
   drained
2 cups sour cream

⅓ cup chili sauce
1 (1¼-ounce) envelope dry onion
   soup mix

- Place salmon in medium mixing bowl. Add sour cream, chili sauce, and soup mix. Stir until well blended. Cover.

- Refrigerate at least 3 hours. Stir.

- Serve with crackers or fresh vegetables. Makes 3½ cups.

Mrs. Bruce H. McCullar (Jennifer)

Hot Tennessee Dip

1 cup chopped pecans
2 teaspoons butter
2 (8-ounce) packages cream cheese, softened
4 tablespoons milk

5 ounces dried beef, minced
1 teaspoon garlic salt
1 cup sour cream
4 teaspoons minced onion

- Preheat oven to 350 degrees when ready to bake.

- Sauté pecans in butter. Reserve.

- Mix other ingredients thoroughly. Place in 1½-quart baking dish. Top with pecans. Chill until serving time. Bake 20 minutes. Serve hot with crackers or small bread sticks.

Variation: Add 2 tablespoons chopped green bell pepper and ⅛ teaspoon red pepper.

Mrs. James R. Ross (Lucy)
Mrs. W. L. Burgess, Jr. (Delores)

Tomato Soup Dip

1 (3-ounce) box lemon gelatin
1 (10¾-ounce) can tomato soup
1 (8-ounce) package cream cheese
1 cup chopped onion

1 cup chopped pecans
1 cup chopped green bell pepper
1 cup mayonnaise

- Sprinkle gelatin over soup and add cream cheese. Cook over low heat, stirring constantly until cream cheese melts and is well blended.

- Remove from heat and add onion, pecans, green bell pepper, and mayonnaise.

- Serve warm with corn chips.

Mrs. George H. Bouldien (Judy)

Tuna Roll

1 (12½-ounce) can white albacore
tuna, rinsed and drained
1 (8-ounce) package cream cheese

1 tablespoon minced onion
½ cup chopped pecans
1 tablespoon dried parsley flakes

• Mix tuna, cream cheese, onion, and pecans. Chill until firm. Roll in ball and
sprinkle with parsley. Serve with crackers. Serves 10 to 12.

Mrs. Joseph W. Graham (Billie Jean)
Mrs. Cecil L. Raines (Ann)

Mexican Tuna Dip

2 (6½-ounce) cans tuna packed in
water, drained
1 (8-ounce) package cream cheese,
softened

1 (8-ounce) jar Picante sauce
1 teaspoon crushed parsley flakes
¼ teaspoon lemon pepper
1 (18-ounce) package corn chips

• Blend first 5 ingredients and chill 30 minutes. Serve with corn chips. Yields 2
cups.

Mrs. Thomas C. Pyron (Maxine)

Layered Taco Dip

2 (10½-ounce) cans jalapeño bean
dip
3 avocados, peeled and mashed
2 tablespoons lemon juice
½ teaspoon salt
¼ teaspoon pepper
1 cup sour cream
1 cup mayonnaise

1 (1¼-ounce) package taco
seasoning mix
5 green onions, chopped
3 tomatoes, diced
8 ounces cheddar cheese, shredded
1 (4-ounce) can black olives
1 (18-ounce) package tortilla chips

• In 13x9x2-inch baking dish or on flat round tray, layer the following ingredients in
order given: bean dip, avocado mixed with lemon juice, salt, pepper, sour cream
mixed with mayonnaise and taco seasoning.

• Top with one layer of each of the following; green onions, tomatoes, cheese, and
black olives.

• Serve with tortilla chips. Serves 12 to 14.

Miss Traci Sherman

Sweet and Sour Sauce

2 tablespoons cornstarch
½ cup water, divided
1 cup brown sugar
1 cup vinegar

½ cup pineapple juice
¼ cup ketchup
1 tablespoon soy sauce
½ teaspoon salt

- Stir cornstarch into ¼ cup water and set aside.

- Combine the other ¼ cup water with sugar, vinegar, pineapple juice, ketchup, soy sauce, and salt in a saucepan and bring to boil.

- Stir in cornstarch mixture and continue stirring until sauce is the consistency of honey.

- May be served warm or chilled. Yields 2½ cups.

Delicious with Baked Chicken Nuggets (see index).

Mrs. Trent G. Wilson (Sherri)

Tangy Dipping Sauce

1 (18-ounce) jar orange marmalade
5 tablespoons Creole mustard or
brown mustard

5 tablespoons prepared horseradish

- Combine all ingredients and mix well. Serve at room temperature. Yields 2½ cups.

Keeps in refrigerator 2 to 3 weeks.

Mrs. Trent G. Wilson (Sherri)

To curl fresh vegetables such as celery and carrots, cut thinly lengthwise and soak in ice water until ready to use.

Beverages and Soups

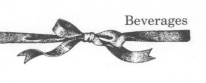

Blue Tail Fly

½ cup blue curaçao
½ cup white crème de cacao

½ gallon vanilla ice cream

• Place curaçao and crème de cacao in blender. Add 2 cups vanilla ice cream and blend. Continue adding vanilla ice cream until you get a thick milk shake consistency. Serve in sherbets or short cocktail glasses. Serves 4.

Nice warm weather dessert drink.

Dr. Charles E. Harbison

Champagne Punch

2 cups lemon juice
2 cups pineapple juice
4 cups strawberry juice (usually takes 5 (10-ounce) boxes frozen strawberries put in blender to make juice)

2 cups sugar, dissolved with about 1½ cups water
1 quart champagne
2 quarts club soda

• Mix first 4 ingredients and pour into punch bowl. Add champagne and club soda.

• Garnish with frozen fruit mold, if desired. Makes about 50 cups.

Mrs. A. G. Baxter (Frances)

Coffee Punch

Instant coffee for 24 cups
½ gallon chocolate ice cream

2 cups whipping cream, whipped

• Make instant coffee.

• Pour hot coffee over ice cream and add whipped cream. Stir together. Serves 30.

Mrs. L. C. Templeton (Virginia)

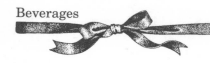

French 75

4 fifths champagne
4 cups brandy

1 (12-ounce) can orange juice,
   thawed, undiluted

- Chill all ingredients. Mix together in punch bowl.
- Doubled recipe will serve 25 people.

Mrs. J. Thomas Cobb (Ann)

Fruit Punch

1 (48-ounce) can cranberry juice
1 (48-ounce) can pineapple juice
1 (48-ounce) can orange juice

½ cup fresh lemon juice
12 (16-ounce) bottles Sprite or 7-up

- Mix juices and pour over ice. Add Sprite or 7-up. Serves 75.

Mrs. Frank J. Hudson (Bettye)

Holiday Punch

1 (12-ounce) can frozen orange juice
1 (6-ounce) can frozen lemon juice
1 (6-ounce) can frozen limeade
5 (12-ounce) cans water

1 cup sugar
1 (46-ounce) can pineapple juice
2 (28-ounce) bottles Fresca

- Mix orange juice, lemon juice, limeade, water, sugar, and pineapple juice.
- Add one bottle Fresca to first punch bowl, then add the second bottle as you replenish punch. Serves 50.

A frozen ring mold makes this more attractive.
Use some of the juices with mandarin oranges, cherries,
sliced strawberries or a fruit to carry out a color scheme.

Mrs. J. Roy Bourgoyne (Helen Ruth)

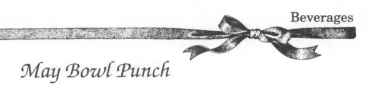

May Bowl Punch

Frozen pineapple ring mold:
24 ounces pineapple juice   1 cup fresh strawberries or peaches

• Combine ingredients and freeze in 4-cup mold.

Punch:
4 cups strawberries or peaches   3 quarts white wine
½ cup sugar   1 quart club soda

• Pour 4 cups desired fruit sprinkled with sugar into punch bowl. Add 1 quart white wine and let stand 12 hours.

• When ready to serve, unmold frozen pineapple mold and place into punch bowl. Add club soda and remaining white wine. Yields 6 quarts or forty-eight 4-ounce cups.

Mrs. Richard J. Reynolds (Anne)

Uncle Henry's Milk Punch

1 cup bourbon   1½ cups sugar
1 cup brandy   5 cups milk
½ cup rum   Grated nutmeg

• Combine ingredients and pour into glasses. Serve with nutmeg sprinkled on top. Yields 8 cups.

Dr. Charles E. Harbison

New Orleans Milk Punch

1 gallon milk   1 fifth bourbon or brandy
1 pound confectioners' sugar   Nutmeg
4 tablespoons vanilla

• Combine all ingredients; mix well.

• Chill or freeze until serving time. If frozen, allow to thaw for awhile before serving and serve as a slush. Sprinkle top with nutmeg.

Mrs. J. Thomas Cobb (Ann)

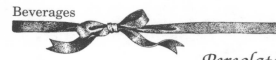

Percolator Punch

2 cups cranberry juice
2½ cups unsweetened pineapple
  juice
½ cup water

⅓ cup brown sugar
1½ teaspoons whole cloves
1½ teaspoons whole allspice
3 sticks cinnamon

- Put cranberry juice, pineapple juice and water in bottom of percolator.

- Place remaining ingredients in basket of percolator and perk as coffee. Serve hot.
  Serves 8.

Mrs. Walter Cooper Sandusky, Jr. (Lois)

Pineapple Cranberry Punch

Ice ring:
32 ounces cranberry juice cocktail

- Freeze in 4-cup mold

Punch:
1 (46-ounce) can pineapple juice
4 cups cranberry juice cocktail

1 quart ginger ale

- Chill all ingredients.

- At serving time, combine and pour into punch bowl over ice ring. Serves 30.

Mrs. Richard C. Harris (Beverly)

Hot Rum Punch

¾ cup sugar
¾ cup water
6 whole cloves
2 cinnamon sticks

8 cups apple cider
4 cups orange juice
½ cup rum

- Simmer first 4 ingredients for 30 minutes. Add cider and orange juice, heating
  thoroughly.

- Add rum just before serving. May also add lemon juice and pineapple juice if
  desired. Serves 20 to 24.

Dr. Phillip Sherman, Jr.

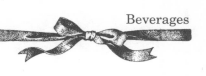

Sangría

Juice of 1 orange
Juice of 1 lemon
¼ cup sugar
⅓ cup cognac
⅓ cup Cointreau (or triple sec)

1 liter red wine (a hearty
 Burgundy)
1 orange, sliced
1 lemon, sliced
12 ounces soda water

- Combine juices and sugar. Add liqueurs, wine, and sliced fruit. With wooden spoon mash fruit. Add soda water. Stir.

- Add ice to pitcher or glasses as preferred.

Mrs. J. Thomas Cobb (Ann)

Strawberry Punch

1 (3-ounce) package strawberry
 gelatin
2 cups sugar
3 cups boiling water
1 (46-ounce) can unsweetened
 pineapple juice

1 (8-ounce) bottle lemon juice
1 (1-ounce) bottle almond extract
2 quarts ginger ale

- Combine gelatin, sugar, and water. Cool. Add juices and almond extract.

- Freeze this mixture in medium size ring mold. Take out 1 hour before serving and add ginger ale. Chip mold with fork to make slushy punch. Serves about 30.

Mrs. Graham H. Morris (Ruth)

Lite Sun Tea

2 family-pack tea bags
1 gallon water
1 individual package Crystal Light
 lemonade

2 packets artificial sweetener

- Let tea steep in sun for 3 hours.

- Add lemonade and sweetener. Stir until well blended. Makes 1 gallon.

Mrs. Phillip Sherman, Jr. (Sandy)

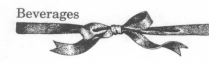

Mint Tea

8 small tea bags
2 quarts boiling water
1 cup sugar
6 to 8 sprigs mint

1 (6-ounce) can frozen lemonade
 concentrate
1 (12-ounce) can pineapple juice

• Pour water over tea bags. Add sugar and mint. Let steep for 30 minutes.

• Remove tea bags and pour mixture into gallon container. Add lemonade (made according to directions on can) and pineapple juice. Serve over ice. Makes approximately 25 cups.

Mrs. H. Franklin Miller (Carolyn)

Tennis Tea

2 family-size tea bags
3 cups boiling water
1½ cups sugar

1 (6-ounce) can frozen limeade
1 (6-ounce) can frozen lemonade
Water to make 1 gallon

• Using a gallon jar, pour boiling water over tea bags. Let stay 10 minutes. Remove tea bags and add remaining ingredients and water to make 1 gallon.

• Serve over ice. Makes about 20 glasses.

Mrs. David B. Fox (Sallie)

Mulled Wine

½ cup sugar
½ cup water
12 whole cloves
2 sticks cinnamon

2 cups orange juice
2 cups pineapple juice
4 cups Burgundy wine

• Mix all ingredients, except wine, and simmer approximately 30 minutes.

• Remove cloves and cinnamon sticks; add wine. Serves 12.

Dr. Charles E. Harbison

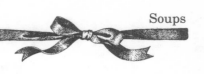

Asparagus Soup

2 (10¾-ounce) cans cream of
  asparagus soup
2 soup cans milk

½ to 1 teaspoon curry powder
4 ounces sliced almonds, toasted

- Mix first 3 ingredients and heat. Do not boil.

- Garnish with toasted almonds and serve as appetizer.

Mrs. J. Roy Bourgoyne (Helen Ruth)

Iced Broccoli Soup

½ cup minced onion
½ cup minced celery
4 tablespoons salad oil
4 tablespoons flour

3 cups chicken broth
1 bunch fresh broccoli, blanched
2 cups half-and-half
Salt and pepper to taste

- Sauté onion and celery in oil. Add flour to make roux. Add broth, stirring until mixture thickens. Cool.

- Put through blender with broccoli. Add half-and-half, salt, and pepper.

- Chill. Serves 8.

Excellent with chicken salad.

Mrs. Richard L. Dixon (Ellen)

Swiss Broccoli Soup

5½ cups whole milk
1 (10-ounce) package frozen
  chopped broccoli
2 tablespoons chopped onion

2 tablespoons butter
1 tablespoon flour
2 cups shredded Swiss cheese
Salt to taste

- Heat milk to simmering. Cook broccoli and onions in milk until tender.

- Melt butter in saucepan, stir in flour, add to milk. Cook and stir 3 minutes.

- Remove from heat, add cheese and salt. Stir until cheese is melted. Serve immediately. Makes 7 to 8 cups.

Mrs. L. C. Templeton (Virginia)

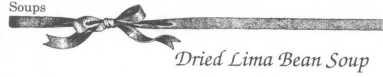

Dried Lima Bean Soup

1 pound dried large lima beans
Water
Chunks of leftover baked ham plus
   bone
4 onions, peeled and quartered
1 clove garlic
2 quarts boiling water

1 tablespoon Worcestershire sauce
4 tablespoons oil
2 tablespoons butter
1 cup canned tomatoes
1 cup finely chopped celery
1 teaspoon salt
Dash grated black pepper

- Soak beans overnight. Remove skins with hands under water.

- Put in 4-quart kettle with all ingredients. Bring to boil, reduce heat and simmer covered 3 to 4 hours. Stir from time to time adding water if necessary. Serves 6 to 8.

Mrs. James L. Wiygul (Lou)

Cheese Soup

4 tablespoons margarine
1 cup water
2 teaspoons instant chicken flavor
   bouillon
⅛ teaspoon onion powder
¼ teaspoon pepper
1 tablespoon cornstarch

2 tablespoons water
1 (10¾-ounce) can condensed
   creamy natural potato soup
1 (5-ounce) can evaporated milk
⅔ cup milk
1 cup shredded sharp cheddar
   cheese

- Combine margarine, water, bouillon, onion powder, and pepper; bring to a boil. Dissolve cornstarch in 2 tablespoons water and stir into boiling liquid.

- Add potato soup, evaporated milk, and milk; simmer 15 minutes. Add cheese and cook slowly until melted. Serves 4 to 6.

Mrs. David R. Libby (Donna)

*S*tart vegetables that grow above the ground in boiling water; start vegetables that grow under the ground in cold water.

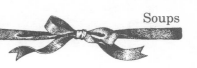

Corn Chowder

½ onion, chopped
2 tablespoons butter
2 tablespoons flour
2 cups whole kernel corn, drained
1 cup diced cooked potatoes

1 (10¾-ounce) can cream of
  mushroom soup
2½ cups milk
Salt to taste
Bacon bits

- Cook onion in butter until done, then add flour.

- Add remaining ingredients and heat thoroughly.

- Top with bacon bits.

Mrs. Kenneth L. Isaacman (Sherry)

Cream of Cucumber Soup (Cold)

3 cucumbers, chopped
½ cup chopped onion, shallots or
  scallions
3 tablespoons butter
6 cups chicken stock
1½ teaspoons light wine vinegar

¼ teaspoon dill weed
4 tablespoons quick cooking farina,
  cream of wheat or minute tapioca
Salt and pepper to taste
1 cup sour cream
Dill or parsley, for garnish

- Sauté cucumbers and onion in butter for 5 minutes.

- Add next 4 ingredients and simmer for 20 to 25 minutes, stirring to keep the
  thickening from sticking. Cool. Purée in blender. Salt and pepper to taste.

- Chill, then add 1 cup sour cream and blend again.

- Garnish with dill or parsley. Makes 7 to 8 cups.

Mrs. Richard J. Reynolds (Anne)

Use ice cube trays to freeze small amounts of stock. Pop out when frozen and store in freezer bags.

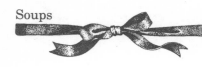

Duck Gumbo

4 large onions
1 bunch celery
¾ cup vegetable oil
6 to 8 mallard or equivalent ducks
1 cup oil
1 cup flour
26 cups water
1 tablespoon salt

¼ teaspoon red pepper
2 to 3 pounds smoked pork link
 sausage
4 cups long grain rice, uncooked
Gumbo filé
1 bunch parsley
2 bunches green onions, chopped

- Chop onions and celery in food processor; sauté in large black skillet in ¾ cup vegetable oil. Remove onions and celery and brown seasoned ducks. Remove ducks and save drippings.

- Prepare a roux by adding oil and flour to drippings in skillet. Cook on medium high heat, stirring constantly, until flour is dark brown (almost burned). Set aside.

- Put roux and water in 12-quart pot and stir until mixture has a smooth consistency. Add onions, celery, ducks with breast down, salt, and red pepper. Cook on low heat until tender, approximately 2 to 3 hours. Do not boil.

- Cook sausage, drain grease, cut into small pieces, add to ducks; allow 2 hours cooking with ducks.

- Remove ducks from pot, pull meat from bones, and return duck meat to mixture. Cook 30 minutes while constantly dipping grease from surface.

- Cook rice according to package directions. Serve gumbo over rice sprinkled with gumbo filé, and garnish with parsley and green onions. Serves 20.

To degrease hot gumbo, add ice cubes to solidify grease,
or float lettuce leaf on top to absorb grease.

Dr. Charles E. Harbison

*N*ever salt heavily at the beginning of stock-making. It will concentrate as it cooks *and be too salty. Wait until you have finished, and then season to taste.*

French Market Soup

1 (16-ounce) package dried 16 bean
  soup
3 quarts water
2 ham hocks
3 to 4 pieces chicken, skin removed
1 (28-ounce) can whole tomatoes

1 large onion, coarsely chopped
1 green bell pepper, chopped
2 cloves garlic
1 tablespoon Tony Chachere's
  Cajun seasoning
1 pound Polish sausage

• Rinse beans and soak overnight.

• Drain beans and add 3 quarts water and ham hocks. Simmer 3 hours covered.

• Add remaining ingredients, except for sausage, and simmer 1½ hours uncovered.
  Before serving, remove meat from ham hocks and chicken bones.

• Sauté sausage and add to beans along with chicken and ham.

Mrs. Michael J. Harty (Kay)

Gazpacho

½ clove garlic
1 (1½-ounce) package Spanish rice
  seasoning mix
1 cup tomato juice
1½ pounds fresh tomatoes
1 medium cucumber, peeled and
  chopped

¼ minced green bell pepper
¼ cup minced onion
2 tablespoons olive oil
3 tablespoons vinegar
1 tablespoon seasoned pepper

• Rub large bowl with garlic clove. Empty seasoning mix into bowl. Add tomato
  juice. Stir well.

• Peel tomatoes, remove core and chop finely. Add tomatoes, cucumber, green bell
  pepper and onion to seasoned tomato juice. Add oil and vinegar. Mix well.

• Cover and chill overnight. Add sprinkle of seasoned pepper. Serves 6.

Mrs. N. Edward Tillman (Ann)

Mallett's Brunswick Stew

1 whole chicken
1 large onion, sliced
3 ribs celery, cut into pieces
Salt, pepper, and garlic powder to
   taste
3½ quarts water

1 (16-ounce) can lima beans
1 (16-ounce) can whole kernel corn
1 (14½-ounce) can stewed tomatoes
½ cup ketchup
3 tablespoons Worcestershire sauce
¾ teaspoon cayenne

- Place chicken, onion, celery, salt, pepper, garlic powder, and water in 5-quart Dutch oven. Boil until meat falls from bone, about 45 minutes.

- Remove all bones and add remaining ingredients. Bring back to boil, reduce heat and simmer for 1½ hours. Serves 8 to 10.

Delicious with cornbread. Very hearty!

Mrs. John Mallett Barron (Doy)

The Very Best Onion Soup

6 large yellow onions
¾ cup butter
2 tablespoons flour
1 tablespoon sugar
4 (10¾-ounce) cans beef bouillon

1 cup red wine
Salt and pepper to taste
Toasted rounds French bread
Gruyère, Swiss or Parmesan
   cheese, grated

- Peel onions and slice thinly, separating the rings.

- Melt butter, add onions, and cook gently, stirring with wooden spoon until rings are golden brown.

- Sprinkle rings with flour and sugar. Stir gently.

- Heat beef bouillon and wine together. Drop rings into this mixture. Stir until soup begins to boil. Lower heat, simmer for 20 minutes. Add salt and pepper.

- Serve with a toasted round of French bread heaped with grated cheese. Serves 6 to 8.

Mrs. June Prichard Robinson

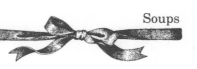

Seafood Bisque

1 (10¾-ounce) can pepper pot soup
1 (10¾-ounce) can cream of celery soup
1 soup can half-and-half
1 teaspoon sugar
Dash garlic powder
Dash paprika
1 or 2 tablespoons chopped parsley
½ package frozen seafood sticks, diagonally sliced

- Mix all ingredients together.

- Heat. Do not boil. Serves 4. Doubled, serves 8 to 10.

The Cookbook Committee

Seafood Gumbo

5 pounds okra, sliced
1 cup plus 2 tablespoons bacon drippings
2 cups flour
8 quarts water
1 stalk celery, chopped
3 or 4 green bell peppers, chopped
4 very ripe tomatoes, chopped
4 onions, chopped
3 or 4 bay leaves, crushed
2 tablespoons garlic powder
2 tablespoons dried chives
2 teaspoons gumbo filé (optional)
2 tablespoons Worcestershire sauce
1½ cups sherry
Salt and Tabasco to taste
5 pounds peeled shrimp
3 (12-ounce) jars fresh oysters
2 (6½-ounce) cans crabmeat
2 pounds cod fillets, cut into pieces
1 bunch green onions with tops, chopped

- Smother okra in 2 tablespoons bacon drippings until all sliminess has gone (about 45 minutes). Set aside.

- Make roux, using 1 cup bacon drippings to 2 cups flour. Stir this mixture over medium heat until very brown, but not scorched. Must stir constantly. Set aside.

- Bring to boil 8 quarts of water. Add smothered okra, roux, celery, green bell peppers, tomatoes, onions, spices, sherry, seasoning, and all juice from the seafood. Bring to a boil. Reduce heat. Keep this barely bubbling for 2 to 2½ hours.

- Forty-five minutes before serving, add seafood and turn up heat a little. Cook 30 minutes. Remove from heat. Sprinkle green onions and tops over the cooked mixture and allow to set at least 15 minutes before serving.

- Ladle into soup bowls and add a scoop of rice. Serve with French bread and a green salad. Serves 20 to 25. Freezes well.

Mrs. William H. McHorris (Jackie)

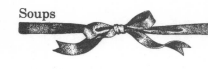

She-Crab Soup

1 (3-ounce) package cream cheese with chives
1 (10½-ounce) can Harris Atlantic She-Crab soup
1 (10¾-ounce) can tomato soup
2 (10¾-ounce) cans cream of celery soup
4 cups milk
Chopped green onions to taste
1 (6-ounce) can lump crabmeat
½ cup sherry

- Mix first 6 ingredients.

- Heat until almost boils.

- Add lump crabmeat and sherry. Serves 8 to 10.

Mrs. Charles E. Harbison (Betty)

Squash Soup

4 to 5 medium yellow squash
2 medium onions
1 large baking potato
1 (10¾-ounce) can chicken broth
1 soup can water
¼ teaspoon ground cumin seed (optional)
1 tablespoon chopped parsley
Salt and pepper to taste
¼ cup butter
Half-and-half cream or milk
Sour cream (optional)

- Thinly slice all vegetables. Place in pan with chicken broth, water, and spices. Cook until tender about 20 to 30 minutes.

- Remove vegetables from broth and purée in blender or food processor. Add butter.

- Add reserved broth and cream until desired thickness is reached.

- Serve hot or cold with spoonful of sour cream. Serves 6.

Mrs. Joe Hall Morris (Adair)

Always simmer soups, never boil them.

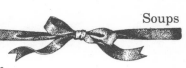

Clear Tomato Soup

¼ cup diced celery
¼ cup diced carrots
¼ cup diced onion
2 tablespoons butter
1 tablespoon parsley
4 cups tomato juice

½ teaspoon white pepper
6 cloves
1 bay leaf
1 teaspoon salt
⅛ teaspoon thyme
2 (10½-ounce) cans beef consommé

- Sauté vegetables in butter. Add remaining ingredients except consommé. Bring to a boil. Cover and simmer 1 hour.

- Strain through a sieve. Add consommé and reheat. Serves 6.

Mrs. Dan Dooley (Jan)

102

Bonnie's Vegetable Soup

1 small green bell pepper, chopped
1 medium onion, chopped
2 tablespoons parsley flakes
½ teaspoon salt
⅛ teaspoon garlic powder
⅛ teaspoon pepper
2 tablespoons butter

2 cups cubed cooked beef
1 (10¾-ounce) can beef broth
1 (10¾-ounce) can old fashioned
    vegetable soup
2 soup cans cold water
1 (15-ounce) can tomatoes, cut up
1 cup shell noodles

- In large saucepan cook green bell pepper, onions, and seasonings in butter until tender. Add remaining ingredients and cook until noodles are done.

- Makes 9 cups.

"A wonderful way to use leftover roast."

Dr. Marion Johnston

103

*A*dd potatoes if soup is too salty, cook a few minutes, and then discard potatoes.

Savory Vegetable Soup

2 packages beef stew meat
2 packages short ribs
Water
2 carrots, diced
2 celery ribs, chopped
1 onion, diced
1 large potato, diced
2 tablespoons sugar
1 (28-ounce) can tomatoes
1 (10¾-ounce) can tomato soup

1 bay leaf
1 teaspoon salt
1 teaspoon pepper
1 (10½-ounce) can whole kernel
   corn
1 (15-ounce) can lima beans
1 (10-ounce) package frozen okra
1 cup uncooked macaroni,
   if desired

- In large soup pot cover meat with water and cook until tender, about 3 hours. Remove bones from short ribs and any fat from stew meat. Add to meat and broth carrots, celery, onion, potato, sugar, tomatoes, soup, bay leaf, salt, and pepper. Cook for 30 minutes.

- Add corn, lima beans, okra, and macaroni. Cook another 30 minutes. May have to add more salt and pepper. Season to your own taste. Serves 16.

Mrs. Phillip Sherman, Jr. (Sandy)

Crème Vichyssoise

5 leeks or spring onions, finely
   chopped (green tops reserved)
1 medium onion, finely sliced
¼ cup sweet butter
5 medium Idaho potatoes, thinly
   sliced
1 quart chicken broth

1 tablespoon salt
2 cups milk
2 cups half-and-half
1 tablespoon Worcestershire sauce
Few drops Tabasco
Celery salt to taste
1 cup whipping cream

- Sauté leeks and onion lightly in butter. Add potatoes, chicken broth, and salt. Boil until potatoes are done.

- Run this through strainer or blender. Add milk and bring to boil; cool.

- Add half-and-half and rest of seasonings and chill.

- Whip cream and add about 1 hour before serving time.

- Chill until ready to serve. Sprinkle each serving with finely chopped green tops. Serves 10 to 12.

Mrs. G. W. Huckaba (Ann)

Salads
and
Dressings

Hawaiian Chicken Salad

4 cups cubed cooked chicken
1 cup diced celery
1 (8-ounce) can sliced water
   chestnuts
1 cup green seedless grapes
1 cup fresh pineapple chunks
½ cup mayonnaise

½ cup sour cream
2 teaspoons curry powder
1 tablespoon soy sauce
Salt and pepper to taste
2 hard-boiled eggs
¼ cup toasted almonds

• Toss chicken, celery, water chestnuts, grapes, and pineapple carefully. Combine mayonnaise, sour cream, and seasonings; mix into tossed ingredients. Add eggs and sprinkle with almonds. Serves 8 to 10.

Mrs. Richard J. Reynolds (Anne)

Shrimp Salad

2 cups cooked chopped shrimp
1 cup finely chopped celery
4 hard-boiled eggs, chopped
2 tablespoons chopped sweet pickle

1 tablespoon finely chopped onion
⅛ teaspoon salt
Mayonnaise to desired consistency

• Mix all ingredients and chill. Serves 5 to 6.

Mrs. A. Joe Fuson (Jean)

Mixed Fruit Deluxe

1 (15¾-ounce) can pineapple
   chunks, drained
1 (11-ounce) can mandarin oranges,
   drained

1 (21-ounce) can peach pie filling
1 (10-ounce) package frozen
   strawberries, thawed
2 bananas, sliced

• Mix all ingredients and chill. Serves 6.

Serve as a salad, dessert, or topping on ice cream.

Mrs. Thomas H. Shipmon (Betty)

Fruit Salad with Tropical Sauce

Salad:

4 cups watermelon balls
2 cups cantaloupe balls
3 kiwis, peeled and sliced
1 cup red grapes

1 cup green grapes
2 cups blueberries
2 peaches, peeled and sliced

- In large bowl combine fruit.

- Refrigerate until chilled. Serve with sauce. Serves 10 to 12.

Sauce:

1 cup sour cream
¼ cup fresh coconut
¼ cup apricot preserves

1 tablespoon dry white wine
½ cup almonds, toasted and
  chopped

- Combine all ingredients in bowl and stir well.

Mrs. William F. Slagle (Shannon)

Fruit Salad with Banana Cream

¼ pound plums
2 navel oranges
2 kiwis
2 ripe pears
1¼ cups (6-ounces) seedless green
  grapes
1¼ cups (6-ounces) seedless red
  grapes

1 pint strawberries, hulled and
  sliced
½ cup sugar
1 ripe banana
1 tablespoon honey
1 cup heavy cream, chilled

- Peel and cut fruit into bite size pieces.

- Layer first 7 ingredients in order as listed. Sprinkle each layer with 1 tablespoon sugar. Cover with plastic wrap and refrigerate overnight.

- Cut banana into chunks and place in food processor with 1 tablespoon honey. Purée until smooth. With processor still running, add 1 cup heavy cream and process 1 minute.

- Serve cream on top of fruit.

- Banana cream may be made 4 hours ahead. Serves 8 to 10.

Mrs. Phillip Sherman, Jr. (Sandy)

Ann's Cranberry Salad

2 cups fresh cranberries
2 cups miniature marshmallows
¾ cup sugar
2 cups diced red delicious apples, unpeeled
½ to ¾ cup seedless green grapes, sliced

½ cup English walnuts, coarsely chopped
1 (8-ounce) can crushed pineapple, drained
¼ teaspoon salt
1 cup whipping cream

- Grind cranberries in blender or food processor until fine. Add marshmallows and sugar. Let mixture stand overnight in refrigerator.

- Combine apples, grapes, walnuts, pineapple, and salt. Mix cranberry mixture with these fruits.

- Whip cream until stiff. Toss all ingredients with whipped cream. Serves 10 to 12.

Wonderful for a holiday buffet.

Mrs. Phillip Sherman, Jr. (Sandy)

Pickled Peach Salad

1 (28-ounce) jar pickled peaches
1 (6-ounce) package lemon gelatin
½ cup water
½ cup orange juice
Juice of 1 lemon

1 (8-ounce) jar white cherries or canned white grapes, drained
⅛ teaspoon salt
1 cup chopped pecans

- Drain and cut peaches, reserving 1 cup juice. Heat juice and dissolve gelatin. Add water, orange juice, and lemon juice. Add fruit. Mix in salt and nuts. Pour into 6-cup ring mold and chill. Serves 6 to 8.

Great with ham.

Mrs. Joe Hall Morris (Adair)

Artichoke Lettuce Salad

1 head romaine lettuce
1 head iceberg lettuce
1 (4-ounce) jar chopped pimentos, drained
1 (10-ounce) can artichoke hearts, drained and diced

1 red onion, thinly sliced
½ to 1½ cups grated Parmesan cheese
⅓ cup white vinegar
½ cup oil
Salt and pepper, if desired

- Wash, drain, and tear lettuce. Do not cut.

- Combine pimentos, artichoke hearts, sliced onion, and cheese with lettuce.

- Combine vinegar and oil; pour over lettuce. Season with salt and pepper. Toss. Cover and refrigerate at least 1 hour. Serves 10 to 12.

Mrs. Ralph E. Knowles, Jr. (Janet)

Charlemagne Salad

Salad:
1 head curly endive
1 head iceberg lettuce

1 head romaine lettuce
1½ cups garlic croutons

- Tear lettuce into bite size pieces and toss with croutons in large bowl.

Dressing:
½ cup olive oil
4 teaspoons minced shallots
2 teaspoons minced garlic
½ cup sherry wine vinegar
2 tablespoons fresh lemon juice

2 tablespoons Dijon mustard
10 ounces Brie cheese, softened, rind removed, and cut into small pieces
Salt and pepper to taste

- Warm oil in large skillet over low heat for 10 minutes. Add shallots and garlic. Cook until translucent. Stir about 5 minutes.

- Blend vinegar, lemon juice, and mustard. Add cheese and stir until smooth. Season with salt and pepper.

- Toss hot dressing with lettuce. Serves 10 to 12.

Mrs. J. Lawrence McRae (Rebecca)

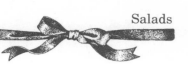

Caesar Salad

3 cloves garlic, pressed
2 tablespoons anchovy paste
1 teaspoon Worcestershire sauce
8 tablespoons olive oil
Freshly ground pepper
2 tablespoons wine vinegar

1 head romaine lettuce, broken into
  pieces
1 egg, boiled 1 minute
1 cup croutons
½ cup freshly grated Parmesan
  cheese

- In wooden bowl mash garlic, anchovy paste, Worcestershire, 1 tablespoon olive oil and pepper. Place in refrigerator until ready to make the salad.

- Add remaining olive oil and vinegar and blend well. Toss dressing with romaine.

- Break egg into salad and toss again. Add croutons and toss. Add cheese to taste. Serves 6 to 8.

Mrs. J. Lawrence McRae (Rebecca)

Guacamole Salad Bowl

Avocado Dressing:
½ cup mashed avocado
1 clove garlic, crushed
1 tablespoon lemon juice
½ teaspoon sugar
½ cup sour cream

½ teaspoon chili powder
⅓ cup salad oil
¼ teaspoon salt
Dash Tabasco

- Beat with beater or blender.

Salad:
½ head iceberg lettuce
½ cup sliced ripe olives
¼ cup chopped green onions
2 tomatoes, cut in wedges

1 cup corn chips
1 (6½-ounce) can tuna, rinsed and
  drained

- Break lettuce and mix with other ingredients.

- Toss lightly with avocado dressing.

Garnish:
½ cup shredded cheddar cheese
Olive slices

Avocado slices

- Serves 6.

Mrs. Justin D. Towner (Ginny)

Avocado Mandarin Green Salad

2 cups iceberg lettuce
2 cups romaine lettuce
2 cups red tipped lettuce

1 (11-ounce) can mandarin oranges, drained
1 large avocado, diced

- Mix and toss above ingredients.

- Delicious when served with poppy seed or vinaigrette dressing. See Index.

Fresh strawberries may be added when in season.

Cookbook Committee

Spinach Layered Salad

Salad:
1 small bunch fresh spinach
½ pound bacon, cooked and crumbled
½ medium onion, thinly sliced
1 (1½-ounce) package slivered almonds

1 (10-ounce) package frozen peas, thawed
1 (8-ounce) can sliced water chestnuts, drained
⅓ head lettuce, torn into bite size pieces to cover

- In 3-quart casserole, layer salad ingredients in order given.

Dressing:
2 cups mayonnaise
1 (1-ounce) package dry ranch dressing mix

Grated Parmesan cheese to cover

- Mix mayonnaise and ranch dressing, then spread over lettuce.

- Sprinkle with Parmesan cheese. Cover with plastic wrap and chill overnight.

- Do not toss before serving. Serves 12.

Mrs. J. Howard McClain (Virginia)

Seven Layer Salad

1 head lettuce, shredded or broken
   into small pieces
1 cup chopped celery
1 green bell pepper, chopped
1 (10-ounce) box frozen green peas,
   cooked and drained

1 pint mayonnaise
2 teaspoons sugar
1 cup grated Parmesan cheese
8 slices bacon, cooked and
   crumbled

- Layer ingredients in serving bowl as listed. Refrigerate overnight or for several hours. Add bacon just before serving. Serves 12 to 14.

Mrs. J. Roy Bourgoyne (Helen Ruth)

Italian Summer Salad

Salad:
1 small head romaine lettuce
½ medium head iceberg lettuce
2 cups spinach leaves
12 mushrooms, sliced

6 Roma tomatoes, diced
18 black olives, sliced
4 ounces cheddar cheese, cubed
4 green onions, sliced

- Prepare ingredients and place in large plastic bag, seal and refrigerate.

Dressing:
½ cup olive or vegetable oil
⅓ cup wine vinegar

1½ teaspoons salt
1½ teaspoons dried oregano leaves

- Prepare dressing, shaking all ingredients in covered jar. Refrigerate.

- Just before serving, shake dressing. Add to salad in bag. Close bag and shake until well coated. Pour salad into serving bowl. Serves 6 to 8.

Mrs. William F. Slagle (Shannon)

Duck and Dried Tomato Salad

Marinade:

½ cup oil drained from 7-ounce jar
  marinated, dried tomatoes
2 tablespoons white wine vinegar
1 clove garlic, minced

⅛ teaspoon Tabasco
⅛ teaspoon Worcestershire sauce
⅛ teaspoon salt
3 teaspoons toasted sesame seed

- Combine all marinade ingredients in food processor or blender and pulse twice. Let flavors blend for several hours.

Salad:

3 cups thin strips medium rare
  roasted duck, skin and fat
  removed
1 cup thin carrot strips
1 cup thin celery strips
1 sweet red pepper, cut into thin
  strips

4 green onions, thinly sliced
½ cup chopped parsley
12 dried tomatoes, cut into strips
Mixed greens

- Place salad ingredients, except for mixed greens, in large bowl and add marinade. Marinate 5 to 10 minutes and toss lightly. Drain and chill.

- Arrange on bed of crisp mixed greens. Serves 4.

May substitute cooked chicken, beef, fish, etc.
It makes a beautiful main dish salad.

Mrs. James R. Wyatt (Mary Kate)

South of the Border Salad

1 pound lean ground round,
  browned, drained, and cooled
1 (1.25-ounce) package El Paso taco
  seasoning mix
1 head lettuce, chopped
3 cups shredded cheddar cheese
1 (15-ounce) can kidney beans,
  rinsed, drained, and chilled

2 medium tomatoes, diced
½ onion or 1 bunch green onions,
  finely chopped
1 (12-ounce) package taco flavored
  Dorito chips, broken
1 (8-ounce) bottle Catalina dressing
Sliced ripe olives (optional)

- Toss all salad ingredients. Add Catalina dressing to taste and garnish with sliced ripe olives, if desired.

- Serve immediately. Serves 6.

Delicious served in pita pockets.

Dr. Beth Harbison

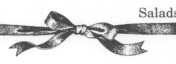

Taco Salad

1½ pounds ground beef
1 teaspoon chili powder
1 teaspoon cumin
1 teaspoon salt
1½ cups chopped onion
1 cup chopped celery

1 cup chopped green bell pepper
3 buds garlic
1 head lettuce, shredded
2 tomatoes, chopped
1 pound Velveeta, melted
1 (10-ounce) can Rotel tomatoes

- Brown first 4 ingredients. Add and sauté next 4 ingredients with beef mixture. Drain.
- After cooling beef mixture slightly, spoon onto bed of lettuce and chopped tomatoes.
- Melt Velveeta, add Rotel tomatoes, and pour over salad. Top with crushed Doritos. Serves 6.

Mrs. James B. Cochran (Linda)

Gazpacho Aspic

2 packages unflavored gelatin
3 cups tomato juice
¼ cup wine vinegar
1 clove garlic
2 teaspoons salt
¼ teaspoon pepper
⅛ teaspoon cayenne
2 large tomatoes, chopped and
  drained
½ cup finely chopped onion

¾ cup finely chopped green bell
  pepper
¾ cup chopped cucumber, drained
½ cup chopped pimento
Salad greens
Hot peppers
Dilled okra
½ cup sour cream
½ teaspoon salt
⅓ cup mayonnaise

- Soften gelatin in 1 cup tomato juice. Heat mixture to simmer. Add remaining tomato juice, vinegar, garlic, salt, pepper, and cayenne. Chill until mixture begins to set. Fold in tomatoes, onion, bell pepper, cucumber, pimento, and pour into 6-cup mold.
- Unmold on salad greens. Surround with peppers and okra if desired. Make dressing from remaining ingredients and spread over top. Serves 8.

Mrs. Richard L. Dixon (Ellen)

Ambrosia Congealed Salad

1 (3-ounce) package orange gelatin
1 cup boiling water
1 cup crushed pineapple, undrained
⅓ cup sugar

1 cup chopped pecans
1 cup mandarin oranges
½ cup flaked coconut
1 cup sour cream

• Dissolve gelatin in hot water. Add pineapple, sugar, and cool.

• Add remaining ingredients and pour into 4 to 5-cup mold. Chill until set. Serves 8.

Mrs. Roy M. Smith (Katherine)

Chicken Cranberry Layer Salad

Chicken Layer:
2 envelopes unflavored gelatin
(softened in ½ cup cold water
over low heat)
1 cup mayonnaise
1 teaspoon salt

3 tablespoons lemon juice
1 cup chopped celery
2 tablespoons chopped parsley
2 cups cooked and chopped chicken
breasts

• Blend all ingredients. Pour into 13x9x2-inch baking dish. Chill until firm.

Cranberry Layer:
1 envelope unflavored gelatin
(softened in ¼ cup cold water
over low heat)
1 (16-ounce) can whole berry
cranberry sauce

1 (9-ounce) can crushed pineapple,
drained
1 tablespoon lemon juice
Nuts (optional)

• Mix all ingredients. Pour over chicken layer. Chill until firm. Sprinkle nuts on top if desired. Serves 10 to 12.

Mrs. James R. Ross (Lucy)
Mrs. Justin D. Towner (Ginny)

Tart Cherry Salad Mold

1 (16-ounce) can tart red cherries
1 (8-ounce) can crushed pineapple
½ cup sugar

2 (3-ounce) packages cherry gelatin
1½ cups ginger ale
½ cup chopped nuts

- Drain fruit and reserve juices.

- In 3-quart saucepan add water to juices to make 1½ cups. Add sugar and bring to a boil. Stir in gelatin until dissolved.

- Remove from heat and stir in fruit and ginger ale.

- Add nuts and pour into 8-cup mold and chill.

Mrs. Stephen Weir (Dottie)

Congealed Asparagus Salad

1 cup cold water
½ cup white vinegar
¾ cup sugar
½ teaspoon salt
2½ envelopes unflavored gelatin
½ cup cold water
1 (10½-ounce) can asparagus
    spears, drained

1 (2-ounce) jar chopped pimentos,
    drained
¾ cup chopped celery
1 teaspoon grated onion
½ cup chopped nuts (optional)

- Heat 1 cup water and vinegar to boiling. Add sugar and salt; stir until sugar is dissolved.

- Mix gelatin in ½ cup water. Add to hot mixture and stir until gelatin completely dissolves.

- Chill until gelatin mixture is slightly thickened. Add asparagus, pimentos, celery, onion, and nuts. Pour into 5-cup mold and chill until firm. Serves 6 to 8.

Mrs. Thomas H. Shipmon (Betty)
Mrs. Chester Lloyd (Betty)

Quick Cranberry Salad

1 (6-ounce) package raspberry
  gelatin
1½ cups boiling water
1 (16-ounce) can whole berry cranberry sauce
1 (8-ounce) can crushed pineapple,
  drained

3 tart apples, diced
3 oranges, peeled and diced
2 celery ribs, diced
½ cup chopped nuts

- Dissolve gelatin in water. Add remaining ingredients and pour into 2-quart mold and chill. Serves 6 to 8.

Mrs. P. D. Miller, Jr. (Greene)

Cucumber Salad

1 (6-ounce) package lime gelatin
2 cups boiling water
1 cup chopped cucumber
1 cup chopped celery
1 cup mayonnaise

1 (20-ounce) can crushed pineapple,
  drained
2 teaspoons onion juice
⅛ teaspoon salt

- Mix gelatin with boiling water. Cool.

- Add remaining ingredients to gelatin mixture.

- Pour into 5-cup mold and chill. Serves 8 to 10.

Mrs. Chester Lloyd (Betty)

Orange Salad

1 (6-ounce) package orange gelatin
1½ cups boiling water
1 (12-ounce) can frozen orange
  juice, undiluted
2 (11-ounce) cans mandarin
  oranges, drained

1 (15-ounce) can crushed pineapple,
  drained
1 cup sour cream

- Dissolve gelatin in boiling water. Add orange juice, oranges, pineapple, and sour cream. Pour into 2-quart mold and refrigerate.

Delicious when served with game.

Mrs. Charles E. Harbison (Betty)

Orange Molded Salad

Salad:
2 (3-ounce) packages orange gelatin
1 cup hot water
1 (15¼-ounce) can crushed pineapple, drained, juice reserved

1 (6-ounce) can frozen orange juice,
thawed
1 cup miniature marshmallows
3 bananas, sliced

- Mix above ingredients except pineapple juice and pour into 13x9x2-inch Pyrex dish. Congeal.

Topping:
1 egg, beaten
½ cup sugar
2 tablespoons flour

1 cup pineapple juice
1 cup whipping cream, whipped

- In saucepan, add slowly to the beaten egg, sugar, flour, and pineapple juice. Cook until custard consistency.

- Cool. Fold in whipping cream and top gelatin salad. Serves 20.

Mrs. Edward J. Weiner (Rochelle)

Raspberry Salad

Salad:
1 (6-ounce) package raspberry
gelatin
2 cups boiling water
2 (10-ounce) packages frozen
raspberries and juice

1 cup applesauce
¼ teaspoon lemon juice

- Dissolve raspberry gelatin in boiling water. Add raspberries, applesauce, and lemon juice; pour into 8-cup salad mold.

Topping:
1 cup sour cream

40 miniature marshmallows

- Mix together and refrigerate overnight. Spread topping on salad before serving.

Dr. Beth Harbison

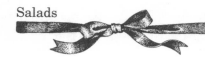

Tuna Salad

2 packages unflavored gelatin
¼ cup water
1 (10-ounce) can mushroom soup
1 cup cottage cheese
1 cup mayonnaise
2 tablespoons grated onion

Juice of ½ lemon
½ cup diced celery
¼ cup diced green bell pepper
2 tablespoons chopped pimento
1 (7-ounce) can tuna, drained
Salt and pepper to taste

- Soak gelatin in water.

- Heat soup. Add gelatin and remaining ingredients.

- Put into 5-cup salad mold. Chill until set; serves 6 to 8.

May also be served with crackers as appetizers.

Mrs. James F. Bigger, Jr. (Pat)

Polynesian Fruit Salad

1½ cups sour cream
¾ cup sugar
⅛ teaspoon salt
2 tablespoons lemon juice
½ cup broken pecans or walnuts

1 (6-ounce) jar maraschino cherries,
   drained and chopped
1 (16-ounce) can crushed pineapple,
   drained
2 large ripe bananas, diced

- Combine sour cream, sugar, salt, and lemon juice. Add nuts, cherries, pineapple, and bananas. Stir just enough to blend evenly.

- Pour into 2-quart mold or muffin tins lined with fluted liners. Place in freezer 4 hours or until firm. Serves 12.

Variation: Add coconut.

Mrs. James E. Sexton (Pat)
Mrs. Warren L. Lesmeister (Carol)

Pineapple Fruit Freeze

1 (21-ounce) can cherry or
strawberry pie filling
1 (14-ounce) can sweetened
condensed milk
1 (13-ounce) container whipped
non-dairy topping

1 (7-ounce) can coconut
1 cup chopped pecans
1 (16-ounce) can crushed pineapple,
undrained

• Mix all ingredients together. Put in individual muffin tins or 13x9x2-inch dish.
Remove from freezer shortly before serving. Serves 10 to 12.

Mrs. Kenneth L. Isaacman (Sherry)

Frosty Peach Salad

1 (10-ounce) package frozen sliced
peaches
1 (3-ounce) package orange gelatin

1 cup boiling water
¼ teaspoon almond extract
2 cups non-dairy whipped topping

• Thaw, drain, and chop peaches, reserving sugar syrup.

• Dissolve gelatin in boiling water. Add water to reserved syrup to make 1 cup, and
combine with gelatin. Add extract and blend well.

• Chill until bowl and mixture are cool (30 minutes). Stir in peaches and topping.

• Freeze in 8-inch square dish or lined muffin tins. Serves 8.

Mrs. Thomas C. Patterson (Margaret)

Frozen Grape Salad

2 (3-ounce) packages cream cheese
2 tablespoons mayonnaise
2 tablespoons pineapple syrup
24 regular marshmallows,
quartered

1 (16-ounce) can pineapple tidbits,
drained
1 cup whipping cream, whipped
2 cups Tokay grapes, halved and
seeded

• Blend softened cream cheese and mayonnaise. Beat in pineapple syrup. Add
marshmallows and pineapple. Fold in whipped cream and grapes.

• Pour into 2-quart dish. Freeze until firm. Makes 8 servings.

Mrs. Joe L. Cannon (Nell)

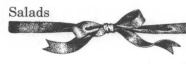

Fruit Salad Delight

16 large marshmallows
1 (20-ounce) can pineapple tidbits,
   drained (reserve 2 tablespoons)
1 (8-ounce) package cream cheese

1 (20-ounce) can fruit cocktail,
   drained
1 cup chopped nuts

- Melt marshmallows in saucepan with reserved pineapple juice, stirring constantly.

- Mash cream cheese and add to marshmallow mixture. Add all fruit and nuts. Serve chilled from the refrigerator or salad may also be frozen. Serves 6 to 8.

Mrs. W. L. Burgess, Jr. (Delores)

Frozen Fruit Basket

1 (16-ounce) can whole berry
   cranberry sauce
1 (8-ounce) can crushed pineapple,
   undrained
1 (8-ounce) carton non-dairy
   whipped topping

1 (8-ounce) carton sour cream
½ cup chopped pecans
3 large ripe bananas
Lettuce leaves

- Mix first 6 ingredients in order listed.

- Spoon into paper-lined muffin tins. Freeze. Remove from tins and put in baggies in freezer.

- Thaw at room temperature 10 to 15 minutes before serving. Arrange on lettuce leaves. Serves 18 to 24.

Mrs. Justin D. Towner (Ginny)

Artichoke-Rice Salad

1 (12-ounce) can artichoke hearts,
   drained
½ to ¾ cup French dressing
1 cup rice, uncooked
2 cups chicken broth
¼ cup diced green onions

¼ cup sliced ripe olives
¼ cup mayonnaise
½ teaspoon dill weed
1 (4-ounce) can sliced water
   chestnuts

- Marinate artichokes in French dressing 3 hours.

- Cook rice in broth, cool. Combine remaining ingredients. Chill. Serves 6 to 8.

Mrs. Walter Cooper Sandusky, Jr. (Lois)

Old Fashioned Potato Salad

6 to 8 medium potatoes, boiled
5 hard-boiled eggs, chopped
½ tablespoon chopped onion
6 candied dilled pickle strips, diced
1 (2½-ounce) jar chopped pimentos, drained

Salt and pepper to taste
½ teaspoon mustard
1 cup mayonnaise

- Boil potatoes until slightly done. Chill 2 hours before removing skin and dicing.

- Combine eggs, onion, pickle, and pimentos. Add to potatoes. Salt and pepper generously. Add mustard and mayonnaise. Chill overnight. Serves 8 to 10.

Mrs. Charles E. Harbison (Betty)

Fresh Broccoli-Cauliflower Salad

Dressing:
1 cup mayonnaise
⅓ to ½ cup sugar

2 tablespoons vinegar

- Mix the above ingredients.

Salad:
1 bunch broccoli, chopped
1 small head cauliflower, chopped
½ cup chopped purple onion
12 slices bacon, cooked crisp and crumbled

2 tablespoons sesame seed
1 cup white raisins

- Chop broccoli and cauliflower with knife, not food processor.

- Mix all ingredients. Add dressing and marinate in refrigerator overnight. Serves 6 to 8.

Mrs. L. Carl Anderson (Maxine)

*P*ut a dry sponge in crisper drawer of refrigerator to absorb moisture.

Creamy Broccoli Salad

Dressing:

¾ cup mayonnaise
¼ cup sugar

3 tablespoons vinegar

• Combine ingredients and set aside.

Salad:

4 cups broccoli flowerets
¼ cup chopped onion
½ cup chopped pecans

1 (8-ounce) can water chestnuts,
　drained and sliced
½ pound bacon, fried crisp

• Mix all ingredients and marinate in dressing.

Mrs. George H. Bouldien (Judy)

Broccoli Oriental Salad

1 large bunch broccoli
1 (7½-ounce) can water chestnuts,
　drained and sliced
1 (4-ounce) can mushrooms,
　drained
½ cup sliced stuffed olives
1 small onion, grated, or 1
　tablespoon chopped green onion

1 cup mayonnaise
1 tablespoon lemon juice
1 teaspoon sugar
2 to 4 strips bacon, cooked, drained
　and crumbled

• Peel stalks of broccoli, splitting larger ones lengthwise.

• Combine remaining ingredients and toss with broccoli. Serves 8.

Mrs. Richard J. Reynolds (Anne)

To prepare lettuce in advance, rinse leaves and drain well. Wrap in a kitchen towel and store in refrigerator until ready to assemble salad.

Calico Vegetable Salad

Salad:

1 (16-ounce) can English peas, drained
1 (16-ounce) can French style green beans, drained
1 (12-ounce) can shoe peg corn
1 (4-ounce) jar pimentos, undrained

1 green bell pepper, finely chopped
1 cup chopped celery
½ cup chopped green onions with tops
1 cup grated carrots (or minced in food processor)

Marinade:

½ cup vegetable oil
½ cup apple cider vinegar
½ cup sugar

⅛ teaspoon each: oregano, parsley, tarragon, and accent

- Bring oil, vinegar, and sugar to boil. Add seasonings and pour over vegetables.

- Refrigerate overnight. Serves 8 to 10.

Delicious served on a bed of shredded lettuce sprinkled with lemon pepper.

Mrs. Lee E. Wilson (Carol)

Corn Slaw

1 (12-ounce) can white shoe peg corn, drained
3 green onions with tops, finely diced
1 tomato, finely diced
½ green bell pepper, finely diced

2 cups chopped cabbage
1 tablespoon sweet pickle relish
3 tablespoons vinegar
3 to 4 tablespoons mayonnaise
Salt and pepper to taste

- Mix corn, onion, tomato, bell pepper, cabbage, and relish.

- Mix vinegar and mayonnaise together. Toss with vegetables and chill. Serves 4 to 6.

Better if made a day ahead. Add more mayonnaise if needed.

Mrs. L. Carl Anderson (Maxine)

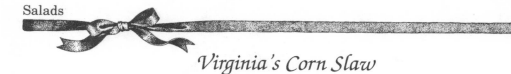

Virginia's Corn Slaw

½ cup sour cream
½ cup mayonnaise
2 teaspoons prepared mustard
4 teaspoons white vinegar
2 teaspoons sugar
½ teaspoon salt
¼ teaspoon pepper

3 (12-ounce) cans white shoe peg corn, drained
4 carrots, finely chopped
2 green bell peppers, seeded and diced
1 cup red onion, chopped (optional)

• Mix well and refrigerate at least 1 hour before serving. Yields 8 to 10 servings.

Mrs. L. C. Templeton (Virginia)

Hot Slaw

1 head red cabbage
2 tablespoons sugar
1 teaspoon salt

½ cup vinegar
½ cup water
2 tablespoons butter, melted

• Preheat oven to 350 degrees.

• Shred cabbage.

• Mix sugar, salt, vinegar, water, and butter. Pour over cabbage and mix.

• Place in large casserole or Dutch oven. Bake 1 hour. Serves 8 to 10. Freezes well.

Great with beef or venison.

Mrs. James L. Wiygul (Lou)

Sweet and Sour Slaw

1 large head cabbage, shredded
1 large onion, sliced into thin rings
¾ cup sugar
1 cup vinegar
1 teaspoon prepared mustard

1 tablespoon sugar
1 teaspoon celery seed
1½ teaspoons salt
1 cup corn oil

• Mix cabbage, onion, and ¾ cup sugar.

• Bring next 5 ingredients to boil. Add corn oil. Bring to second boil and pour over cabbage mixture.

• Let stand overnight. Serves 10.

Mrs. N. Edward Tillman (Ann)

Sauerkraut Salad

1 (16-ounce) jar sauerkraut
½ cup cauliflower
½ cup broccoli
3 tablespoons chopped green onion

½ cup chopped sweet red pepper
½ cup sugar
½ cup vinegar

- Rinse sauerkraut and mix with vegetables.

- Mix sugar and vinegar. Heat until sugar is melted. Pour over sauerkraut and vegetable mixture.

- Chill in refrigerator at least 24 hours. Keeps several days in refrigerator. Serves 6 to 8.

Mrs. J. W. Breazeal (Sue)

Savory Summer Salad

2 (16-ounce) cans shredded kraut
1 cup chopped celery
1 large onion, chopped
1 green bell pepper, chopped
1 (8-ounce) can water chestnuts, thinly sliced

1 (4-ounce) jar pimentos, drained and chopped
¼ cup wine vinegar
½ cup corn oil
1 cup sugar

- Rinse and drain kraut. Combine all vegetables in large bowl.

- Combine vinegar, oil, and sugar in saucepan; bring to boil. When sugar is dissolved, pour hot mixture over vegetables. Refrigerate. Serve cold. Makes 2 quarts.

Best if made a day or two ahead of time.

Mrs. Michael J. Harty (Kay)

Cucumber-Onion in Marinade

1 cucumber, sliced
1 onion, sliced
1 pod dried red pepper, seeded and crushed

3 tablespoons sugar
½ cup cider vinegar
1 teaspoon salt
½ teaspoon pepper

- Combine all ingredients. Toss and stir. Serves 2 to 4.

Keeps approximately 3 days in refrigerator.

Mrs. Richard L. Dixon (Ellen)

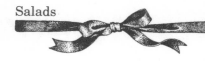

Italian Tomatoes

1 (16-ounce) bottle Italian dressing
¼ teaspoon garlic powder
½ teaspoon soy sauce

1 teaspoon oregano
5 to 6 fresh medium tomatoes,
  quartered

- Mix first 4 ingredients. Pour over tomatoes. Store covered in refrigerator. Serves 10 to 12.

Mrs. Frank J. Hudson (Bettye)

Fire and Ice Tomatoes

¾ cup vinegar
¼ cup water
1½ teaspoons mustard seed
1½ teaspoons celery salt
½ teaspoon salt
4½ teaspoons sugar

⅛ teaspoon red pepper
⅛ teaspoon black pepper
6 large tomatoes, cut in quarters
1 onion, cut in slices and separated
1 green bell pepper, cut in strips

- Combine vinegar, water and seasonings and boil 1 minute.

- Pour over vegetables and chill several hours. Will keep 2 to 3 days. Serves 8.

Mrs. Charles E. Harbison (Betty)

Broccoli Mold

2 envelopes unflavored gelatin
½ cup cold water
1 (10½-ounce) can condensed
  consommé
1 teaspoon beef stock base
Dash Tabasco
1¾ teaspoons salt

5 teaspoons Worcestershire sauce
6 teaspoons lemon juice
¾ cup mayonnaise
2 (10-ounce) boxes frozen chopped
  broccoli (cooked as directed)
4 hard-boiled eggs, grated

- Dissolve gelatin in cold water.

- Heat to boiling: consommé, beef base, Tabasco, salt, Worcestershire, and lemon juice. Add gelatin and cool.

- Fold in mayonnaise, broccoli, and eggs. Pour into 6-cup mold and chill. Serves 10.

Mrs. Dan T. Meadows (Amy)

Crunchy Vegetable Salad

2 envelopes unflavored gelatin
1¾ cups water, divided
¼ teaspoon salt
¼ teaspoon white pepper
⅓ cup vinegar
¾ cup sugar
1 cup shredded cabbage

2 cups chopped celery
1 (7-ounce) jar pimentos, diced
1 cup grated carrots
1 (8-ounce) can green peas, drained
1 cup chopped pecans
Salad greens

- Soften gelatin in 1 cup water and set aside.

- Combine ¾ cup water, salt, pepper, vinegar, and sugar in saucepan. Bring to boil and remove from heat. Add softened gelatin mixture, stirring until dissolved. Chill until slightly thickened.

- Stir cabbage, celery, pimento, carrots, peas, and nuts into thickened gelatin. Spoon mixture into lightly oiled 6-cup mold.

- Chill until firm and unmold on salad greens. Serves 8 to 10.

Mrs. Ernest H. Sigman, Jr. (Doris)

Marinated Vegetable Medley

1 (17-ounce) can small green peas, drained
1 (16-ounce) can French style green beans, drained
1 onion, thinly sliced

1 green bell pepper, chopped
1 (8-ounce) can water chestnuts, drained and sliced
1 cup sliced celery, cut diagonally

- Combine vegetables in bowl; set aside.

Marinade:
½ cup vegetable oil
¾ cup vinegar

¾ to 1 cup sugar
1 teaspoon salt

- Mix marinade ingredients and heat thoroughly until sugar is dissolved. Pour over vegetables; chill overnight. Drain before serving. Keeps for a week in refrigerator. Serves 6 to 8.

When making a large quantity,
use fewer onions and water chestnuts in proportion.

Mrs. J. Roy Bourgoyne (Helen Ruth)

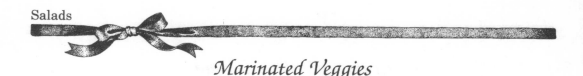

Marinated Veggies

1 bunch cauliflower flowerets
1 bunch broccoli flowerets
5 medium carrots, cut in strips
3 ribs celery, chopped

1 to 2 pounds fresh mushroom
  buttons
2 cucumbers, sliced
2 to 3 squash, sliced

- Cook first 3 vegetables slightly and drain. Add celery and mushrooms.

Marinade:
1½ cups oil
3 cups tarragon vinegar
½ cup sugar
⅛ teaspoon garlic powder

1 tablespoon prepared mustard
1½ teaspoons salt
2 teaspoons tarragon leaves
Pepper to taste

- Mix marinade ingredients and pour over vegetables. Chill overnight. Add squash and cucumber. Serves 10 to 12.

Mrs. Justin D. Towner (Ginny)

Pasta Salad

1½ cups small elbow macaroni
3 tablespoons olive oil
Juice of 1½ lemons, freshly
  squeezed
Celery salt and lemon pepper to
  taste
2 carrots, sliced

½ green bell pepper, chopped
2 green onions, chopped
2 hard-boiled eggs, chopped
½ to ¾ cup mayonnaise
Parsley
Paprika

- Cook macaroni. Rinse and drain. Combine macaroni, oil, lemon juice, celery salt, and lemon pepper.

- Combine with vegetables and cover. Chill salad and prepared eggs.

- When ready to serve, combine eggs and mayonnaise; gently mix. Garnish with parsley and paprika. Serves 6.

The longer it marinates, the better it is.

Mrs. Clyde Jennings (Zana Lee)
— Submitted in her memory by her daughter.

Rainbow Pasta Salad

12 ounces rainbow rotini
1 tablespoon chicken bouillon
  granules
4 cups broccoli flowerets
1 (15-ounce) can white chicken,
  or 1 cup cooked chopped chicken
  breasts

½ cup stuffed olives, sliced
2 cups lite mayonnaise

- Cook pasta according to package directions, adding chicken bouillon granules to pasta water. Drain and cool pasta.

- Fold in remaining ingredients and chill. Serves 8 to 10.

Mrs. David R. Libby (Donna)

Tiny Ring Macaroni Salad

2 packages tiny salad macaroni
  rings
9 hard-boiled eggs, sliced
2 (13-ounce) cans tuna
2 cups chopped celery
¼ onion, finely chopped (optional)

2 (17-ounce) cans English peas,
  drained
4 ounces cheddar cheese, cubed
1 (4-ounce) jar pimento olives,
  sliced
Salt and pepper to taste

- Cook macaroni. Chill in cold running water and drain.

- Mix all ingredients; add salt and pepper to taste.

Dressing:
½ to ¾ cup mayonnaise

2 tablespoons prepared mustard

- Mix well, toss with salad mixture. Serves 18.

Diced ham or shrimp may be substituted for tuna.

Mrs. Richard C. Harris (Beverly)

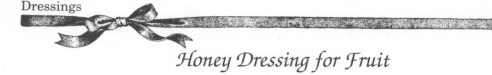

Honey Dressing for Fruit

½ cup orange juice
1 tablespoon fresh lemon juice
1 tablespoon lime juice

2 tablespoons honey
½ cup chopped pecans

• Mix all above in jar and shake. Pour over any combination of fruit with pecans added.

Fruit suggestions:

• Pineapple chunks, mandarin oranges, diced apples, halved seedless grapes, sliced bananas

Mrs. Thomas C. Patterson (Margaret)

Kum Bac Salad Dressing

1 cup mayonnaise
½ cup ketchup
½ cup chili sauce
1 teaspoon mustard
½ cup salad oil
1 tablespoon horseradish

¼ teaspoon Tabasco
1 teaspoon paprika
Juice of 1 lemon
1 medium onion, grated
1 teaspoon black pepper
2 tablespoons water

• Blend all ingredients thoroughly; store in refrigerator. Makes 3 cups.

Mrs. Joe Hall Morris (Adair)

Pineapple Dressing

Juice from 1 (20-ounce) can sliced
    pineapple
2 tablespoons butter, softened
2 tablespoons flour

1 egg
¾ cup sugar
⅛ teaspoon salt
½ cup whipping cream, whipped

• Heat pineapple juice. Blend butter and flour and add to juice.

• Stir in well beaten egg, sugar, and salt. Cook until thick.

• When cool, fold in whipped cream. Serve with mixed fruit or congealed salad. Makes about 2 cups.

Mrs. Joe Hall Morris (Adair)

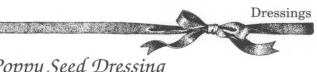

Easy Poppy Seed Dressing

⅓ cup honey
⅓ cup frozen limeade concentrate

⅓ cup vegetable oil
2 tablespoons poppy seed

• Mix all ingredients in jar and shake well.

• Serve over fresh or canned fruit. Makes 1 cup.

Mrs. Frank J. Hudson (Bettye)

Poppy Seed Dressing

1½ cups sugar
2 teaspoons dry mustard
⅔ cup vinegar
2 teaspoons salt

2 cups oil
2 teaspoons poppy seed
2 teaspoons grated onion

• Mix together first 5 ingredients. Beat until thick.

• Add poppy seed and onion. Mix well. Serve over fruit salad. Makes 3 cups.

Mrs. J. B. Edmonds (Jeanne)

Herb Vinaigrette Dressing

½ cup olive oil
¼ cup lemon juice
½ cup chopped fresh basil

1 tablespoon chopped fresh parsley
1 teaspoon pepper

• Combine all ingredients. Mix thoroughly. Yields 1 cup.

Mrs. Lyle E. Muller (Mary)

Doy's French Dressing

1 cup sugar
1 cup ketchup
¾ cup vinegar
1½ cups vegetable oil

3 teaspoons salt
½ teaspoon paprika
⅛ teaspoon black pepper
1 large onion, chopped

• Mix all ingredients. Chill. Makes 1 quart and keeps indefinitely in refrigerator.

Mrs. John Mallett Barron (Doy)

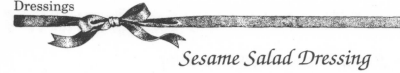

Sesame Salad Dressing

1 cup oil
¼ cup sugar
1 teaspoon salt
1 teaspoon dry mustard

2 green onions, chopped
⅓ cup red wine vinegar
1 teaspoon sesame seed

• Blend first 5 ingredients until smooth.

• Add wine vinegar and sesame seed right before serving.

Good on red-tip lettuce, avocado and mandarin oranges.

Mrs. Thomas H. Shipmon (Betty)

Tarragon Salad Dressing

1 tablespoon dried tarragon
⅓ cup lemon juice
¾ cup olive oil

¼ teaspoon fresh or dried parsley
Salt and pepper to taste

• Combine all ingredients. Mix thoroughly. Makes 1 cup.

Cookbook Committee

Shrimp Salad Dressing

2 cups Hellmann's mayonnaise
1 onion, grated
1 teaspoon garlic salt
2 hard-boiled eggs, chopped

1 kosher dill pickle, chopped
1 teaspoon dry mustard
Juice of 1 lemon
¼ teaspoon chopped parsley

• Combine all ingredients. Mix well. Yields enough dressing for 3 to 4 pounds boiled shrimp.

Mrs. Phillip Sherman, Jr. (Sandy)

Breads
and
Muffins

Apple Strudel

Filling:

1 (15-ounce) can sliced apples, drained and sliced again
½ (10-ounce) bottle maraschino cherries, drained and sliced
1 (7-ounce) package coconut
1 (6-ounce) can crushed pineapple, drained well
½ (15-ounce) box white raisins
¾ cup chopped nuts
1 tablespoon lemon juice
1½ to 2 teaspoons cinnamon
¾ cup sugar

- Mix filling ingredients together. Set aside.

Dough:

2 cups flour
½ teaspoon baking powder
1 teaspoon salt
¼ cup cooking oil
1 egg
2 to 3 tablespoons hot water
Sugar
Cinnamon

- In large bowl, place dry ingredients and make well in center. Beat oil and egg together; pour into well. Mix and add few tablespoons water until dough is consistency to knead. Knead several times.

- Cover bowl with towel and set in warm oven so dough will be easier to handle.

- Preheat oven to 350 degrees.

- Divide dough into 3 sections. Roll ⅓ of warm dough on floured surface until about ⅛-inch thin. Oil heavily with pastry brush, and sprinkle with sugar and cinnamon.

- Put ⅓ filling in center of dough and fold one edge over the filling. Tuck in ends. Brush with oil, sprinkle with cinnamon and sugar. Continue rolling like jelly roll. Oil top and sprinkle again.

- Place seam side down on cookie sheet. Slice ⅓ way through into small slices. Pierce top of each slice with knife.

- Bake 30 minutes until brown. Remove from cookie sheet and slice each piece all the way through.

Mrs. Danny Weiss (Saralyn)

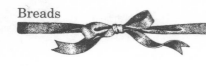

Angel Biscuits

2 envelopes active dry yeast	3 teaspoons baking powder
1 teaspoon sugar	1 teaspoon salt
¼ cup warm water	¼ cup sugar
(110 to 115 degrees)	1 cup Crisco
5 cups flour	2 cups buttermilk
1 teaspoon baking soda	

- Mix yeast, 1 teaspoon sugar, and water. Let stand 10 minutes.

- Sift together flour, soda, baking powder, salt and sugar.

- Cut in shortening with pastry blender until mixture resembles coarse meal. Add buttermilk and yeast, stirring until well mixed. Knead lightly.

- Place in bowl. Cover. Put in refrigerator until needed.

- Roll out on lightly floured surface, cut with biscuit cutter and place on baking sheet, leaving a little space between each biscuit.

- Place in warm spot for 1 hour to rise.

- Bake in 400 degree oven until lightly browned, 18 to 20 minutes.

Dough will keep in refrigerator for 2 days if well covered.

Mrs. Winfield Dunn (Betty)

Bachelor's Dream Doughnuts

2 cups vegetable oil	Confectioners' sugar
1 can refrigerator biscuits	

- Heat oil to constant 375 degrees.

- Cut hole in center of each biscuit with top from oil bottle.

- Drop biscuits in hot oil and cook for 45 seconds. Turn over and cook an additional 45 seconds. Lift out and drain.

- Dip hot doughnut in confectioners' sugar or a mixture of granulated sugar and cinnamon.

- Serve hot and impress your friends!

Dr. J. Roy Bourgoyne

Buttermilk Biscuits

2 cups flour
2 teaspoons baking powder
1 teaspoon salt

¼ teaspoon baking soda
¼ cup shortening
¾ cup buttermilk

- Preheat oven to 450 degrees.

- Mix flour, baking powder, salt, and soda in bowl. Cut in shortening with pastry blender until mixture resembles coarse meal. Add buttermilk and stir with fork until all flour is moistened.

- Place dough on lightly floured waxed paper. Knead six times lightly.

- Roll dough to ½-inch thickness. Cut with biscuit cutter and place on ungreased baking sheet.

- Bake 10 minutes or until brown. Yields 12.

Cookbook Committee

Plantation Coffee Cake

½ cup shortening
¾ cup sugar
1 teaspoon vanilla
3 eggs
2 cups flour
1 teaspoon baking powder

1 teaspoon baking soda
1 cup sour cream
6 tablespoons margarine, softened
1 cup brown sugar, firmly packed
2 teaspoons cinnamon
1 cup chopped nuts

- Preheat oven to 350 degrees.

- Cream shortening, sugar, and vanilla thoroughly. Add eggs, one at a time, beating well after each addition.

- Sift flour, baking powder, and soda together. Add to creamed mixture alternately with sour cream, blending well after each addition.

- Spread ½ of batter in a 10-inch tube pan that has been greased and lined on the bottom with waxed paper.

- Cream margarine, brown sugar, and cinnamon together. Add nuts and mix well.

- Dot batter in pan evenly with ½ of nut mixture. Cover with remaining batter and dot with remaining nut mixture.

- Bake about 50 minutes. Cool cake 10 minutes. Remove from pan.

Mrs. Ernest H. Sigman, Jr. (Doris)

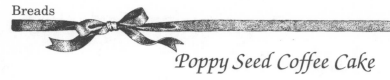

Poppy Seed Coffee Cake

1 package vanilla cake mix
1 (3¾-ounce) package vanilla
  instant pudding
4 eggs

1 cup sour cream
½ cup vegetable oil
½ cup sherry
¼ cup poppy seed

- Preheat oven to 350 degrees.

- Combine all ingredients and pour into greased and floured 10-inch bundt pan. Bake 50 minutes.

Glaze:
1½ tablespoons milk
1 tablespoon margarine
1 tablespoon orange juice

1¼ cups confectioners' sugar
½ teaspoon grated orange rind

- Heat milk, margarine, and orange juice until margarine melts. Stir in sugar and orange rind. Pour over warm coffee cake.

Mrs. Charles E. Harbison (Betty)

Easy Cornbread

1 cup flour
¼ cup sugar
4 teaspoons baking powder
¾ teaspoon salt

1 cup yellow cornmeal
2 eggs, beaten
1 cup milk
¼ cup shortening, melted

- Preheat oven to 425 degrees.

- Sift together flour, sugar, baking powder, and salt. Stir in cornmeal. Add eggs, milk, and shortening; beat in mixer 1 minute. Do not overbeat.

- Pour into greased 8x8x2-inch baking pan. Bake 20 to 25 minutes or until golden brown. Serves 8.

Mrs. P. D. Miller, Jr. (Greene)

Colonial Cornbread

1 cup self-rising cornmeal
2 eggs
1 cup sour cream

1 cup cream style corn
½ cup melted shortening

- Preheat oven to 400 degrees.

- Combine first 4 ingredients, mixing well.

- Heat shortening in 10-inch iron skillet. Pour hot shortening into cornmeal mixture and mix well.

- Return mixture to hot skillet and bake 30 minutes.

Mrs. Roy M. Smith (Katherine)

Corn Light Bread

2 cups cornmeal
¾ cup sugar
½ teaspoon baking soda
1 teaspoon baking powder

½ cup flour
2 cups buttermilk
1 teaspoon salt
2 tablespoons shortening, melted

- Preheat oven to 350 degrees.

- Combine all ingredients. Stir until lightly mixed. Pour into greased 9x5x3-inch loaf pan. Bake 1 hour. Slice when cool.

Mrs. John Mallett Barron (Doy)

Corn Pones

2 cups white stone-ground
  cornmeal
2 teaspoons baking powder
¼ teaspoon baking soda
2 teaspoons salt

2 teaspoons sugar
½ cup boiling water
2 tablespoons Crisco, melted
1 egg, beaten
½ cup buttermilk

- Preheat oven to 425 degrees.

- Mix dry ingredients; add boiling water and shortening. Stir beaten egg into buttermilk and pour into mixture.

- Heat greased cookie sheet. Make 8 mounds of batter. Bake 20 minutes. Makes 8 corn pones.

Dr. P. D. Miller, Jr.

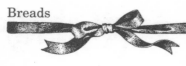

Mexican Cornbread

2 cups cornmeal
1 teaspoon salt
½ cup flour
½ teaspoon baking soda
2 teaspoons baking powder
1 large onion, chopped
½ cup salad oil

4 jalapeño peppers, chopped
2 cups grated cheddar cheese
2 eggs
1 (11-ounce) can whole kernel corn, drained
1 cup sour cream

- Preheat oven to 400 degrees.

- Combine cornmeal, salt, flour, soda, and baking powder in a large bowl and mix well.

- Add remaining ingredients and bake 45 minutes in greased 9x9x2-inch pan. Serves 8.

Mrs. Peggy Sadler

Spoon Bread

3 cups milk
1 cup cornmeal
3 tablespoons butter
1 teaspoon sugar

1 teaspoon salt
3 egg yolks, slightly beaten
3 egg whites, beaten until stiff but not dry

- Preheat oven to 350 degrees.

- Heat milk, gradually add cornmeal, and cook 5 minutes until thickened mush, stirring constantly. Cool slightly. Add butter, sugar, salt, and slightly beaten egg yolks.

- Fold in beaten egg whites. Pour into greased 2-quart casserole. Bake 45 minutes. Serves 6.

Mrs. P. D. Miller, Jr. (Greene)

To prevent sticking and to make a crisp crust, heat greased pan in oven before adding spoon bread batter.

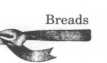

Easy Monkey Bread

**1 (25-ounce) package frozen
parkerhouse rolls**

¼ cup butter, melted

- Preheat oven to 375 degrees when ready to bake.

- Thaw frozen rolls. Cut each roll in half. Dip each piece in melted butter. Arrange pieces in 10-cup bundt or tube pan. Allow to rise until doubled or about 3 hours. Bake 18 to 20 minutes until brown.

Variation: Add garlic powder or Parmesan cheese to melted butter.

Mrs. James F. Bigger, Jr. (Pat)

Joann's Broccoli Muffins

**1 (10-ounce) package frozen
chopped broccoli**
**1 (8½-ounce) package corn muffin
mix**

4 eggs
½ cup margarine, melted
¾ cup cottage cheese
1 onion, chopped

- Preheat oven to 425 degrees.

- Cook broccoli according to package directions. Drain and mash. Mix with remaining ingredients.

- Pour mixture into small greased muffin tins. Bake 10 to 12 minutes or until toothpick comes out clean.

- Yields 54 small muffins.

Mrs. Phillip Sherman, Jr. (Sandy)
Mrs. James F. Bigger, Jr. (Pat)

If paper liners are used, remove muffins from pan to cool. Leave unlined muffins in pan for 5 minutes, then remove.

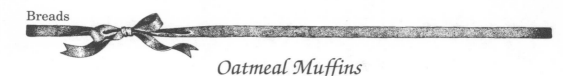

Oatmeal Muffins

1 cup oatmeal
1 cup buttermilk
1 egg
½ cup brown sugar
½ cup oil

1 cup flour
½ teaspoon salt
½ teaspoon baking soda
1 teaspoon baking powder
½ cup nuts or raisins (optional)

- Preheat oven to 400 degrees.

- Soak oatmeal in milk for 5 minutes. Add egg, sugar, and oil.

- Mix together flour, salt, soda, baking powder, and nuts (if used), and add to oatmeal mixture. Batter will be lumpy.

- Fill 12 greased muffin cups. Bake 15 minutes.

Mrs. P. D. Miller, Jr. (Greene)

Piña Colada Muffins

1 (18-ounce) box yellow cake mix
1 teaspoon coconut extract
1 teaspoon rum extract

1 cup flaked or shredded coconut
½ cup chopped walnuts
1 cup crushed pineapple, drained

- Preheat oven to 350 degrees.

- Prepare cake mix in mixer bowl following package directions. Add other ingredients. Mix 1 minute.

- Grease tins or line with paper cups. Fill ¾ full. Bake 15 minutes. Yields 60 miniature muffins.

Cookbook Committee

Party Muffins

1 cup margarine
1 cup sour cream

2 cups self-rising flour

- Preheat oven to 450 degrees.

- Melt margarine and cool slightly. Add sour cream and stir (don't beat), into flour. Spoon into small greased muffin tins. Bake 10 minutes. Yields 24 muffins.

Mrs. J. Roy Bourgoyne (Helen Ruth)

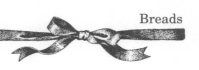

Plum Muffins

2 cups self-rising flour
2 cups sugar
3 eggs
1 cup oil
2 (4½-ounce) jars plum baby food

1½ teaspoons cinnamon
½ teaspoon cloves
½ teaspoon nutmeg
½ cup chopped nuts

- Preheat oven to 350 degrees.

- Mix above ingredients and pour into 18 large greased muffin cups. Bake 15 minutes.

Dr. Beth Harbison

Apricot Bread

1 cup dried apricots, chopped
1 cup warm water
1 cup sugar
2 tablespoons margarine, melted
½ cup orange juice concentrate

2 cups flour
2 teaspoons baking powder
¼ teaspoon baking soda
⅛ teaspoon salt
1 cup chopped pecans

- Preheat oven to 325 degrees.

- Soak apricots in warm water, drain excess water and reserve. Stir in sugar, margarine, ¼ cup reserved juice, and orange juice concentrate.

- Combine flour, baking powder, soda, and salt. Add to apricot mixture. Blend in nuts. Let mixture stand for 20 minutes.

- Bake in greased and floured 9x5x3-inch loaf pan 1 hour and 15 minutes.

Mrs. Justin D. Towner (Ginny)

To make lighter muffins, put greased pans into the oven for a few moments before pouring in batter.

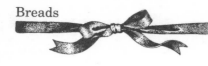

Banana Bread

½ cup margarine
1 cup sugar
2 eggs

1 teaspoon baking soda
2 cups flour
3 ripe bananas

- Preheat oven to 350 degrees.

- Cream margarine and sugar. Add eggs. Fold in dry ingredients.

- Whip bananas until light and add to batter.

- Bake in greased 9x5x3-inch loaf pan for 1 hour.

Variations: 1 cup chopped nuts

1 cup seedless raisins

1 cup finely chopped dates

Mrs. Ernest H. Sigman, Jr. (Doris)
Mrs. Phillip Sherman, Sr. (Barbara)

Blackberry Jam Banana Bread

¾ cup butter
1 cup sugar
3 bananas
2 eggs, well beaten
1 (12-ounce) jar seedless blackberry
  jam

1 teaspoon baking soda
2 cups flour
¾ cup chopped pecans

- Preheat oven to 350 degrees.

- Cream butter and sugar. Mash bananas and add to mixture. Add eggs and jam.

- Combine soda and flour and add to mixture. Blend in nuts. Pour into greased 9x5x3-inch loaf pan. Bake 1 hour.

Mrs. Charles E. Harbison (Betty)

Blueberry Lemon Tea Cake

1 cup blueberries
1 tablespoon flour
½ cup margarine
1 cup sugar
2 eggs

½ cup milk
1⅔ cup flour
1½ teaspoons baking powder
¼ teaspoon salt
1 teaspoon grated lemon peel

- Preheat oven to 350 degrees.

- Toss berries with 1 tablespoon flour and set aside.

- Cream margarine and sugar until light and fluffy. Beat in eggs one at a time. Add milk and dry ingredients until just combined. Fold in berries and lemon peel.

- Bake in greased and floured 9x5x3-inch loaf pan for 60 to 70 minutes.

Glaze:
¼ cup confectioners' sugar

¼ cup fresh lemon juice

- While cake is cooling, combine sugar and lemon juice and heat to boiling. Remove cake after 10 minutes from pan. Prick top and sides and brush with glaze.

Mrs. John Winford (Sherrye)

Date Nut Loaf

2 teaspoons baking soda
½ cup hot water
2 cups chopped dates
½ cup margarine
2 cups sugar

2 eggs, beaten
3 cups flour
1 cup chopped nuts
1 teaspoon vanilla

- Preheat oven to 325 degrees.

- Sprinkle soda and pour water over dates. Set aside.

- Cream margarine and sugar; add eggs and mix well. Add date mixture. Beat in flour, nuts, and vanilla. Bake in greased and floured 10-cup tube pan 1 hour to 1 hour and 15 minutes. Serves 18.

Good with cream cheese.

Mrs. June Prichard Robinson

Boston Brown Bread

1 cup water
¾ cup raisins
2 teaspoons baking soda
2 cups sugar
½ cup margarine or butter

2 eggs
4 cups flour
1 teaspoon salt
1 teaspoon vanilla
1 cup English walnuts, chopped

- Add water to raisins and cook until plump, 5 to 10 minutes. Cool, then add soda and mix very well.

- Preheat oven to 375 degrees.

- Cream sugar and butter. Add eggs, flour, salt, and vanilla. Mix well.

- Dust nuts with small amount of flour and add to creamed mixture alternately with raisin mixture.

- Spoon into 5 or 6 greased 20-ounce cans, filling half full. Bake 45 minutes to 1 hour until toothpick comes out clean.

- May use small orange juice cans for smaller loaves. Bake these 30 minutes. Slice to desired thickness. Serve with softened cheese or flavored butter.

Mrs. Phillip Sherman, Jr. (Sandy)

Bourbon Nut Bread

8 eggs, separated
3 cups sugar, divided
2 cups butter
3 cups sifted flour

½ cup bourbon
2 teaspoons vanilla
2 teaspoons almond extract
1 cup chopped pecans

- Preheat oven to 350 degrees.

- Beat egg whites until soft peaks form. Gradually add 1 cup of the sugar and continue beating until stiff peaks form. Set aside.

- Cream butter with remaining sugar, add egg yolks one at a time, beating well after each addition. Add flour in thirds alternately with bourbon, mixing well. Stir in vanilla, almond extract, and pecans.

- Gently fold in egg whites. Pour into 3 well greased, 9x5x3-inch loaf pans. Bake 1 hour.

This bread freezes well.

Mrs. Frank J. Hudson (Bettye)

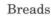

Kate's Cream Cheese Braids

1 cup sour cream	2 envelopes active dry yeast
½ cup sugar	½ cup warm water
1 teaspoon salt	2 eggs, beaten
½ cup butter, melted	4 cups flour

- Heat sour cream over low heat. Stir in sugar, salt, and butter. Cool to lukewarm.

- In large bowl sprinkle yeast over warm water, stirring until dissolved. Add sour cream mixture, eggs, and flour. Mix well. Cover tightly and refrigerate overnight.

- Divide dough into 4 equal parts. Roll out each part on a well floured board into a 12x8-inch rectangle. Make cream cheese filling.

Filling:

2 (8-ounce) packages cream cheese	1 egg, beaten
¾ cup sugar	2 teaspoons vanilla
⅛ teaspoon salt	

- Combine cream cheese, sugar, and salt in mixing bowl. Add egg and vanilla. Mix well.

- Divide filling and spread equally on each piece of dough. Roll up as a jelly roll beginning at long side. Place seam side down on greased cookie sheet. Pinch each roll at 2-inch intervals about two-thirds of the way through dough to resemble a braid.

- Cover and let rise in a warm (85 degrees) draft-free place until doubled. Bake at 375 degrees 12 to 15 minutes. Spread with glaze while warm.

Glaze:

2 cups confectioners' sugar	2 teaspoons vanilla
4 tablespoons milk	

- Combine all ingredients and mix well. Spread over braids. Makes 4 loaves.

Mrs. Phillip Sherman, Jr. (Sandy)

Your bread will be soggy if you leave it in the pan to cool. And do not package hot.

Libby's French Pastry Log

Pastry:
¾ **cup butter**   2 **tablespoons water**
1½ **cups flour**

- Cut butter into flour. Add water. Mix to form pastry. Divide into three balls. Roll each ball like a "snake" until 18-inches long. Press middle of roll with thumb to form a cavity.

Filling:
½ **cup butter**   1 **cup flour, sifted**
1 **cup water**   2 **eggs**
1 **teaspoon almond extract**

- Preheat oven to 350 degrees.

- Put butter into water. Bring to boil. Remove from heat and add almond extract and flour. Beat well by hand. Add eggs one at a time. Mix well.

- Using all of the filling mixture, spoon into cavity of pastry roll. Bake 55 minutes.

Icing:
16 **ounces confectioners' sugar**   1 **teaspoon vanilla**
3 **tablespoons butter**   **Chopped pecans for garnish**
2 **tablespoons milk**

- Combine ingredients and drizzle on pastry while still warm.

- Sprinkle immediately with chopped pecans.

Mrs. Phillip Sherman, Jr. (Sandy)

To glaze the top of pastry, brush with slightly beaten egg white and 1 tablespoon water before baking.

Lemon Nut Bread

⅓ cup margarine, melted
1 cup sugar
2 eggs
½ teaspoon almond extract
½ teaspoon lemon extract

1½ cups flour
1 teaspoon baking powder
½ cup milk
2 teaspoons grated lemon peel
½ cup chopped nuts

- Preheat oven to 350 degrees.

- Cream margarine and sugar. Add eggs and beat well. Add almond extract, lemon extract, flour, baking powder, milk, lemon peel, and chopped nuts.

- Pour into greased and floured 9x5x3-inch loaf pan. Bake 1 hour and 10 minutes.

Glaze:
¼ cup confectioners' sugar

Juice of 1 lemon

- Mix confectioners' sugar and lemon juice. Spoon over bread that has cooled.

Mrs. Frank J. Hudson (Bettye)

All-Bran Refrigerator Rolls

1 cup shortening
¾ cup sugar
1 cup all-bran cereal
1½ teaspoons salt
1 cup boiling water
2 envelopes active dry yeast

½ teaspoon sugar
1 cup lukewarm water
   (110 to 115 degrees)
2 eggs, well beaten
6½ cups flour

- In large mixing bowl combine shortening, sugar, bran, and salt. Add boiling water and allow to stand to cool.

- Combine yeast, sugar, and water and allow to stand 10 minutes.

- Add eggs to bran mixture and then add yeast mixture.

- Add ½ flour and beat well. Add remaining flour and beat until smooth. Cover and place in refrigerator.

- When ready to use, take out of refrigerator and make into rolls. Clover leaf rolls may be made with three balls of dough in a muffin tin. Allow to rise 2 to 3 hours covered with cloth.

- Bake in preheated 400 degree oven for 12 to 15 minutes. Yields 72.

- Keeps 6 weeks in refrigerator.

Mrs. Frank J. Hudson (Bettye)

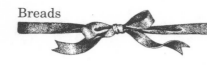

Anybody's Rolls

1 envelope active dry yeast
⅔ cup lukewarm
   (105 to 115 degrees) water
1 cup milk, scalded
⅓ cup shortening

½ cup sugar
1 egg, beaten
4 cups self-rising flour
2 tablespoons margarine, melted

- Dissolve yeast in ⅔ cup lukewarm water. Set aside 10 minutes.

- Scald milk. Place shortening and sugar in bottom of large bowl; add hot milk to dissolve shortening and sugar. Cool to lukewarm. Add 1 beaten egg and yeast mixture. Add flour 1 cup at a time. Dough will be sticky. Roll out on floured board to ¼-inch thickness; cut with 2-inch biscuit cutter. Melt margarine in 13x9x2-inch baking dish. Dip each roll in melted margarine, fold in half, and place in dish. Let rise 1½ hours. Bake in preheated 400 degree oven 15 minutes or until golden brown.

- If you wish to refrigerate dough after it is made, grease sides of bowl and top of dough; cover and refrigerate as long as a week. You may either pinch off amount needed, allow to warm to room temperature and roll out; or roll out all of dough. Yields 36 rolls.

Mrs. Richard J. Reynolds (Anne)

Jeanne Craddock's Rolls

1 cup sugar
1 cup shortening
1 cup boiling water
2 envelopes active dry yeast
¼ cup lukewarm water (110 to 115
   degrees)

1 cup cold water
2 eggs
1½ teaspoons salt
6 cups flour
Vegetable oil
1 cup butter, melted

- Add sugar and shortening to boiling water. Cool in mixing bowl.

- Add yeast that has been mixed with lukewarm water. Add cold water, eggs, and salt. Add flour 2 cups at a time.

- Place dough in bowl and rub top with vegetable oil. Refrigerate overnight.

- Sprinkle flour on counter. Divide dough into 3 parts. Roll out each part until ¼-inch thick. Cut with round biscuit cutter, dip each roll in melted butter, and fold in half with butter on inside. Place on cookie sheet side by side fairly close together.

- Let rise 2½ hours until double in size. Bake in preheated 400 degree oven 10 to 15 minutes. Watch closely. Rolls are ready when golden brown. These rolls freeze beautifully. Cut cooking time in half, cool, and package for freezing. Yields 60 rolls.

Mrs. Phillip Sherman, Jr. (Sandy)

Pocketbook Rolls

2 envelopes active dry yeast
½ teaspoon sugar
¼ cup lukewarm water (110 to 115 degrees)
1 cup milk

1 egg
2 tablespoons sugar
2 tablespoons shortening
1 teaspoon salt
3½ cups flour

- Combine yeast, sugar, and water; allow to stand 10 minutes.

- Scald milk and cool to lukewarm.

- In large bowl, beat egg and add milk, sugar, shortening, salt, and yeast mixture.

- Mix in flour 1 cup at a time with electric mixer on low speed until all flour is moistened. Cover and allow to rise in warm (85 degrees) draft-free place 1 hour or until doubled.

- Roll dough on floured surface to ¼-inch thickness and cut with biscuit cutter. Add ¼ teaspoon butter or margarine to center of each roll and fold in half. Place on greased cookie sheet and allow to rise 45 minutes. Bake in preheated 400 degree oven 20 minutes. Yields 36.

Cinnamon Buns:
- After dough rises the first time, roll to ¼-inch thickness, brush with 2 tablespoons melted margarine or butter, and spread with a mixture of ½ cup sugar, 1½ to 2 teaspoons cinnamon, ⅓ cup raisins, and ⅓ cup nuts.

- Roll up as for jelly roll. Using a thread slice into 1-inch pieces. Place face side down on greased baking sheet and allow to rise for 1 hour.

- Bake in preheated 375 degree oven 15 minutes. Cool slightly. Frost with mixture of 1½ cups confectioners' sugar, 2½ tablespoons milk, and ¼ teaspoon vanilla.

Mrs. P. D. Miller, Jr. (Greene)

Cut unbaked cinnamon rolls by slipping a sewing thread under uncut whole roll and crossing ends of thread to cut rolls to desired thickness.

For plump raisins soak them overnight in sherry or orange juice.

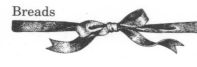

Sally Lunn Bread

2 envelopes active dry yeast
½ teaspoon sugar
¼ cup lukewarm water (110 to 115 degrees)
1 cup milk

½ cup shortening
4 cups flour, divided
⅓ cup sugar
2 teaspoons salt
3 eggs, beaten

- Combine yeast, sugar, and water; allow to stand 10 minutes.

- Heat milk and shortening to 120 degrees, shortening won't melt. Allow to cool.

- In mixing bowl, blend 1⅓ cups flour, sugar, salt; add milk and yeast mixtures. Mix with electric mixer on low speed 1 minute.

- Add beaten eggs and ⅔ cup flour; mix well. Add 1 cup flour, mix well, and add remaining cup flour.

- Cover bowl with cloth and allow to rise in a warm (85 degrees) draft-free place 1 hour and 15 minutes or until doubled.

- Beat dough down in electric mixer and put dough in greased 10-cup bundt pan. Cover pan and allow to rise 30 minutes or until doubled. Bake in preheated 350 degree oven 30 minutes or until top is brown.

Mrs. P. D. Miller, Jr. (Greene)

Ann's Dill Bread

1 package active dry yeast
¼ cup warm water
1 cup creamed cottage cheese
2 tablespoons sugar
1 teaspoon instant onion
1 tablespoon butter, melted

2 teaspoons dill seed
1 teaspoon kosher salt
¼ teaspoon baking soda
1 egg
2¼ to 2½ cups flour, sifted

- Mix thoroughly dry yeast and warm water. Set aside.

- Heat cottage cheese to lukewarm.

- Combine next 7 ingredients in large bowl and mix together with yeast and cottage cheese. Gradually add flour; may need to mix by hand.

- Cover and let rise in a warm place for one hour until doubled in size. Punch dough down and place in 2-quart greased Pyrex baking dish, oblong or round. Let rise a second time about 20 to 30 minutes or until doubled.

- Bake in preheated 350 degree oven 35 to 45 minutes, until brown on top. Brush with butter and sprinkle kosher salt on top.

Mrs. Phillip Sherman, Jr. (Sandy)

Best Coffee Can Dill Bread

1 package active dry yeast	3 tablespoons sugar, divided
½ cup warm water (110 to 115 degrees)	1 (13-ounce) can evaporated milk
⅛ teaspoon ground ginger	1 teaspoon salt
1 tablespoon dill	2 tablespoons salad oil
	4 cups flour

- Dissolve yeast in warm water in large mixing bowl. Blend in ginger, dill, and 1 tablespoon of sugar. Allow to stand in warm (85 degrees) draft-free place until bubbly, about 15 minutes. Stir in remaining 2 tablespoons sugar, milk, salt, and salad oil.

- On low speed of mixer beat in 1 cup of flour at a time. Beat well after each addition.

- Divide dough in half and place in two well greased 1 pound coffee cans. Cover with plastic lids. Let stand in warm place for 45 to 60 minutes until the plastic lids pop off.

- Bake in preheated 350 degree oven for 45 minutes. Brush tops with butter.

- When preparing to serve, slice, butter, wrap in foil, and reheat. Serves 20.

Dough may be frozen in cans. Allow to thaw and rise before baking.

Mrs. J. Roy Bourgoyne (Helen Ruth)

Because flour varies in its absorbency, sprinkle the last measurement into dough mixture so that you can adjust the prescribed quantity. Dough has absorbed enough flour when it pulls away from sides of bowl.

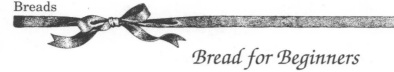

Bread for Beginners

1 envelope active dry yeast
¼ teaspoon sugar
1¼ cups very warm water (110 to
   115 degrees), divided
1 teaspoon sugar

2 tablespoons corn oil
1 teaspoon salt
3½ to 4 cups bread flour or
   unbleached flour

- Dissolve yeast and ¼ teaspoon sugar in ¼ cup water. Cover with plastic wrap. Set aside 5 minutes.

- Pour yeast mixture in 1 cup of very warm water. Add oil and mix well. Combine sugar, salt, and flour. Add to yeast mixture 1 cup at a time. Place dough in well greased bowl. Let rise until doubled in oven that has been warmed for 5 minutes and turned off.

- Punch down with fist. Let dough rest on counter for 20 minutes with bowl inverted over it. Place in greased 9x5x3-inch loaf pan or 9-inch round pan.

- Place pan in warm oven until doubled. Brush top with cold water. Bake in pre-heated 350 degree oven 30 minutes. Remove from pan immediately. Makes 1 loaf.

Mrs. James G. Sousoulas (Sophie)

Have all ingredients for bread at room temperature.

Allow dough to rise in bowl that is not metal.

Bread Bountiful

3 envelopes active dry yeast
1 cup very warm water
4 tablespoons sugar
½ cup flour
2 cups milk
2 tablespoons salt
3 tablespoons Crisco

4 tablespoons margarine
3 eggs, well blended in blender
1 cup water
10 to 10½ cups Pillsbury bread flour
1 egg, beaten
1 tablespoon water

- Place yeast, warm water, sugar, and flour in glass or ceramic bowl which is at least twice the size of these combined ingredients. They will foam and rise quickly. Set aside 5 minutes.

- Scald milk. Add salt, Crisco, margarine, beaten eggs, and water.

- Pour in mixer with dough hook and gradually add flour, one cup at a time. Continue kneading with dough hook until all flour has been used. Dough will be sticky so coat hands generously with Crisco and knead with your hands. This makes dough easily manageable. Too much flour makes bread very dense and heavy.

- Grease large ceramic bowl. Place dough inside and lightly grease top of dough; place plastic wrap on top. Cover bowl with cloth towel; turn oven to warm for 5 minutes, turn off, and place bread in warmed oven.

- Let rise until doubled. Punch down and let dough rest 20 minutes on counter with bowl inverted over it.

- Divide dough in 3 sections. Shape in loaves and place in greased 9x5x3-inch pans. Brush tops with mixture of beaten egg and water.

- Bake in preheated 400 degree oven 5 minutes. Turn oven down to 350 degrees and continue baking 30 minutes. Remove from pan immediately. Makes 3 loaves.

Variation: May omit eggs. If so, leave out 1 cup of flour.

Mrs. James G. Sousoulas (Sophie)

Sour Dough Bread

Starter:

1 envelope yeast
1 cup lukewarm water (105 to 115 degrees)

¾ cup sugar
4 tablespoons instant potato flakes

- Dissolve yeast in warm water in glass container; add sugar and potato flakes and mix well. Cover loosely and let stand 24 hours at room temperature.

- Refrigerate 3 to 5 days.

- On fourth or fifth day remove from refrigerator and add bread feeder.

Bread Feeder:

⅔ cup sugar
3 tablespoons instant potato flakes

1 cup warm water

- Add sugar, potato flakes, and water to bread starter. Stir and let stand 24 hours at room temperature.

- Use 1 cup of regulated starter to make bread.

- Put remaining starter in refrigerator until next feeding. (After initial feeding, starter must be fed every 3 to 5 days. Mix well and let stand at room temperature 8 hours or more. Stir and remove 1 cup starter. Make bread with this starter, give it to a friend, or discard it. Return remaining starter to refrigerator until next feeding.

Sour Dough Bread:

1 cup starter
¼ cup sugar
½ cup corn oil
1 tablespoon salt
1½ cups lukewarm water (105 to 115 degrees)

1 envelope active dry yeast (optional)
6 cups bread flour

- To 1 cup starter, add sugar, oil, salt, and warm water. Add yeast if desired. Add flour, 1 cup at a time, mixing well.

- Put dough in a large greased bowl and brush top with oil. Cover lightly with plastic wrap and leave on counter for about 8 hours.

(continued on next page)

- Punch down with fist and knead well 5 to 10 times. If using 9x5x3-inch greased pans, divide dough into 3 parts. If using 6x3x2-inch greased pans, divide dough into 6 parts.

- Let rise for 6 to 12 hours. Bake on bottom rack of preheated 350 degree oven 30 to 45 minutes.

Starter may be frozen 1 month if
bread maker needs a break or is going on a trip.

Dr. J. Roy Bourgoyne

Whole Wheat Bread

1 envelope active dry yeast	6 tablespoons honey
½ teaspoon sugar	2 teaspoons salt
¼ cup warm water (110 to 115 degrees)	2 cups lukewarm water
	1 egg
6 tablespoons vegetable oil	6 cups whole wheat flour

- Mix yeast, sugar, and warm water. Let stand 10 minutes.

- In large mixing bowl combine oil, honey, salt, and water. Stir in egg and yeast. Add 3 cups flour. Add remaining 3 cups flour. Stir until all flour is wet.

- Turn out on well floured bread board and knead. Dough is very wet, so work in some flour while you knead until dough is elastic. You can't knead too long (at least 5 minutes), but you can work in too much flour so scrape away the flour on the board after dough becomes elastic. Put dough in bowl, cover, and allow to rise 1 hour or until double.

- Stir down and turn on bread board and allow to rest while you grease three 9x5x3-inch pans available in disposable aluminum.

- Knead at least 5 minutes. Divide into 3 parts and knead more as you shape into loaves. Place in well greased pans and gently wipe top of loaves with damp cloth.

- Allow to rise 1 hour or until double. Bake in preheated 350 degree oven 30 to 35 minutes or until top is brown and will "thump" hollow. Turn out of pan to cool.

Mrs. James W. Clark (Carolyn)

Bread Sculptures

A simple, yet dramatic, way to carry out a theme or to complement or highlight a presentation. Simpler even than making dough "from scratch" is buying frozen bread dough; let thaw, then begin design. Make a paper draft of shape first to get an idea of what volume of dough is required. Always use a half inch layer of dough shaped to desired sculpture, then embellish on top of shape. Let rise only 20 minutes. More rising will distort shape.

Harvest Sheaf

2 packages active dry yeast
4½ cups lukewarm (110 to 115 degrees) milk
2 tablespoons salt

2 tablespoons shortening
12 cups flour
2 egg yolks, beaten
2 tablespoons water

- Dissolve yeast in milk, salt, and shortening. Let stand 10 minutes in warm place until frothy.

- Add this liquid to 12 cups flour; mix to form firm dough. Knead in mixer with dough hook for 2 to 3 minutes; or knead with hands on lightly floured surface for 10 minutes.

- Shape dough into ball and place inside large oiled paper bag. Allow to rise for 3 hours or until doubled.

- Knead two minutes or until firm. Divide into halves. Roll half the dough to ½-inch thickness and shape to cover your paper draft for sheaf. Combine egg yolks and water to make wash. Brush dough with wash.

- The remaining half of dough will be used for embellishment on top of base. Roll the dough to ½-inch thickness. Cut 20 thin strands for stalks and two 14-inch strands for ties around sheaf. Use French tin "tearshape" cutter to cut wheat grains. Cover base with grains. Brush on egg wash.

- Let rise 20 minutes. Bake at 350 degrees 40 to 45 minutes until brown.

Thanksgiving Sunday tradition in the Church of England.

Dr. Richard L. Dixon

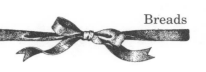

Grape Cluster

**Use harvest sheaf dough or frozen
dough**

- Roll half the dough to ½-inch thickness and shape to cover your paper draft. Brush with egg wash.

- Roll remaining half of dough to ½-inch thickness. Cut leaf shapes, then cut several strands of dough, and roll strands to make tendrils. Roll marble size grapes.

- Brush egg wash on leaves, tendrils and grapes. Continue to pile grapes to make cluster and brush with egg wash as you complete each layer.

- Let rise 20 minutes. Bake at 350 degrees 40 to 45 minutes until brown.

Dr. Richard L. Dixon

Billy's Rye Bread

3 cups sifted flour
2 envelopes active dry yeast
¼ cup cocoa powder
1 tablespoon caraway seed
2 cups water
⅓ cup molasses

2 tablespoons margarine or butter
1 tablespoon sugar
1 tablespoon salt
3 to 3½ cups rye flour
Vegetable oil

- Combine flour, yeast, cocoa, and caraway seed in large mixing bowl until well blended.

- Combine water, molasses, butter, sugar, and salt in saucepan and heat until warm (110 to 115 degrees), stirring to melt butter. Add to first mixture. Beat at low speed with electric mixer for ½ minute, scraping sides of bowl constantly. Beat at high speed 3 minutes.

- By hand, stir in enough rye flour to make a soft dough. Turn onto floured surface and knead 5 minutes until smooth. Cover and allow to rest 20 minutes.

- Punch down and divide dough in half; shape each half into round loaf. Place loaves on greased baking sheets or greased 8-inch pie plates, and brush surface of loaves with vegetable oil. Slash tops of loaves with knife.

- Allow to rise until double for 45 to 60 minutes in warm place.

- Bake in preheated 400 degree oven 25 to 30 minutes. Remove from pan to wire racks to cool.

Dr. Billy W. McCann

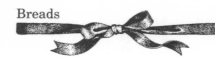

Khashapuri

Filling:

2 pounds Muenster cheese,
  shredded
2 tablespoons butter, softened

1 egg
2 tablespoons ground coriander

- Blend together until thoroughly mixed.

Dough:

2 envelopes active dry yeast
¼ cup lukewarm (110 to 115
  degrees) water
1 tablespoon sugar

1 cup lukewarm milk
½ cup butter, softened
2 teaspoons salt
4 cups flour

- Dissolve yeast in water and sugar. Let stand 10 minutes in warm place until frothy.

- Combine milk, butter, salt, and flour in a mixer with dough hook. Add yeast mixture and beat for 2 minutes. Cover and let rise until doubled or 1 hour.

- Preheat oven to 400 degrees.

- Roll dough on floured surface into a 22-inch circle. Add filling to center. Bring edges of dough toward the center to enclose the filling. Twist dough into a knot.

- Place in greased 10 to 12-inch pie pan and bake 40 minutes. Cool 15 minutes before cutting.

*Filled breads are perfect for brunches or light snacks
or a hearty accompaniment for soups or salads.*

Mrs. Richard L. Dixon (Ellen)

A good bread knife is essential for neat slices without tearing up the loaf.

Steamed Buns

Filling:
1 cup cold water
2 tablespoons cornstarch
½ cup any variety chutney

2 tablespoons hoisin sauce
1 cup ground pork or barbecue or ham

- Combine cold water and cornstarch. Add remaining ingredients and bring to a boil. Cool completely.

Dough:
2½ cups flour
3½ teaspoons baking powder
3 tablespoons sugar
½ teaspoon salt
2 tablespoons lard, softened

½ teaspoon white vinegar
½ cup lukewarm (110 to 115 degrees) water
Sesame oil

- Combine flour, baking powder, sugar, and salt. Cut lard into dry ingredients with pastry cutter or wooden fork.

- Add vinegar to water and pour into flour mixture. Blend and shape into smooth ball; let rest 30 minutes.

- Divide dough into 9 pieces; roll each piece into 4-inch circles. Place heaping teaspoon of filling in center. Pinch edges of dough circles together enclosing filling. Place balls (now buns) pinched edges down on waxed paper. Brush with sesame oil.

- Put ½-inch water in bottom of Dutch oven, add steamer, and place balls on steamer. Steam 20 minutes. May be served immediately or refrigerate and steam again 5 to 10 minutes before serving. Makes 9 buns.

Mrs. Richard L. Dixon (Ellen)

If you let bread rise too long, loaves will have holes.

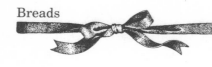

Stuffed Bread

Loaf French bread
¼ cup butter
1 clove garlic, minced
2 tablespoons sesame seed
¼ cup sour cream
1 cup shredded Monterey Jack
 cheese

1 cup grated Parmesan cheese
1 can artichoke hearts, drained and
 chopped
1 cup shredded cheddar cheese

- Preheat oven to 350 degrees.

- Cut French bread in half lengthwise. Pull bread out of center in small chunks.

- Melt butter, sauté garlic, and brown sesame seed. Add bread chunks.

- Combine sour cream, Monterey Jack cheese, Parmesan cheese, and artichoke hearts. Add to bread mixture and put into loaf. (May be frozen at this point.)

- Sprinkle cheddar cheese on top and bake 30 minutes.

Mrs. Kenneth L. Isaacman (Sherry)

Fruity Cream Cheese Spread

1 (3-ounce) package cream cheese,
 softened
1 tablespoon orange juice

2 teaspoons confectioners' sugar
½ apple, peeled and grated

- Mix cream cheese and orange juice. Add other ingredients. Blend. Makes ½ cup.

Mrs. Warren L. Lesmeister (Carol)
Mrs. Thomas C. Patterson (Margaret)

Strawberry Butter

½ cup butter
1½ cups confectioners' sugar

3 to 4 tablespoons mashed fresh
 strawberries

- Mix all ingredients together.

This is wonderful on homemade rolls.

Mrs. Frank J. Hudson (Bettye)

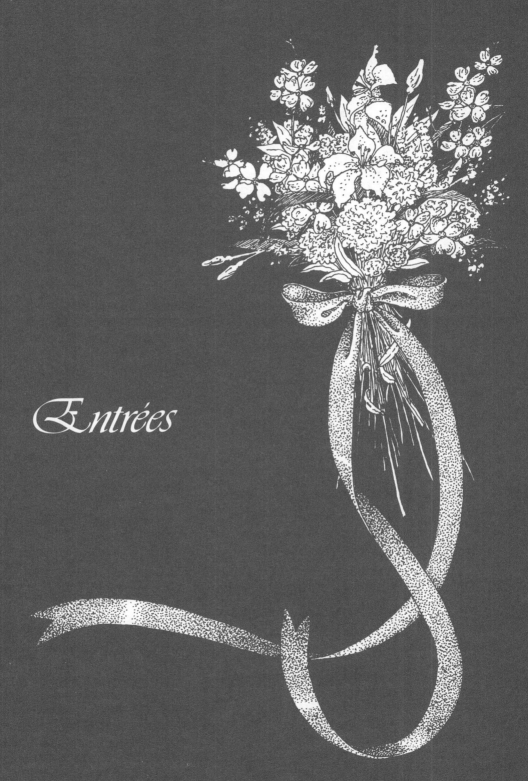

Entrées

Baked Brisket

4 to 6 pound beef brisket
1 (10¾-ounce) can golden
 mushroom soup
1 envelope dry onion soup mix

3 tablespoons Worcestershire sauce
1 teaspoon lemon pepper
¼ to ½ teaspoon garlic powder
1 bay leaf

- Preheat oven to 250 degrees.

- Place brisket in baking pan, fat side up.

- Mix remaining ingredients and spread over meat.

- Cover pan tightly with heavy foil. Bake 6 to 7 hours.

- Slice thin, diagonally across the grain.

I often bake brisket at night. Put brisket in oven at bedtime.
In the morning it's done. It makes wonderful gravy.

Mrs. J. Roy Bourgoyne (Helen Ruth)

Mary Ann Ward's Barbecued Brisket

6 to 8 pound beef brisket, fat
 removed
Onion powder
Garlic salt
Celery salt

2 teaspoons sugar
Worcestershire sauce
2 to 3 drops liquid smoke
¾ cup brown sugar
1 (18-ounce) bottle barbecue sauce

- Rub both sides of meat with onion powder, garlic salt, celery salt, sugar, Worcestershire sauce, and liquid smoke. Refrigerate overnight (fat side up) in foil-lined roasting pan. Cover with foil.

- Preheat oven to 250 degrees and bake brisket 8 hours.

- Remove from oven, open foil and drain off drippings.

- Mix brown sugar and barbecue sauce and pour over meat.

- Return to oven with foil open and bake at 350 degrees for 1 hour. Can be served hot or cold. Serves 12.

Mrs. Stephen Weir (Dottie)

Gourmet Beef Tenderloin

4½ pound beef tenderloin
Salt and pepper to taste

1 cup butter, melted
2 cups hearty Burgundy wine

- Preheat oven to 450 degrees.

- Season tenderloin with salt and pepper. Roll tenderloin in melted butter to coat all sides. Place in shallow baking pan. Pour remaining butter and wine over meat.

- Bake, uncovered, 15 minutes.

- Remove from oven and slice into desired thickness.

- When ready to serve, return meat to oven and cook an additional 15 minutes. Serve immediately. Tenderloin will be cooked to medium-rare doneness.

Dr. Robert Ducklo

Company Eye of the Round

4 pound eye of the round roast or
beef tenderloin

Lemon pepper

- Preheat oven to 450 degrees.

- Season meat liberally with lemon pepper.

- Bake for 5 minutes per pound. Turn oven off. Leave in unopened oven for 2½ hours.

Sauce:
2 tablespoons margarine
2 cups fresh mushrooms
2 tablespoons finely chopped onion
½ cup sherry

1 (10¾-ounce) can beef consommé
Dash pepper
2 tablespoons flour
1 tablespoon melted margarine

- Melt 2 tablespoons margarine in skillet. Sauté mushrooms and onions. Add sherry and cook 2 minutes.

- Add consommé and pepper. Simmer 3 to 5 minutes.

- Mix flour with 1 tablespoon melted margarine. Add to sauce and stir until thickened. Serves 8 to 10 people.

Mrs. Charles E. Harbison (Betty)

Eye of Round Roast

3 to 3½ pound eye of the round roast

Cavenders' dry Greek seasoning

- Preheat oven to 350 degrees.

- Coat roast well with Greek seasoning.

- Wrap in foil and bake 30 minutes per pound.

Mrs. Joe Hall Morris (Adair)

Marinated Eye of Round Roast

4 pound eye of round roast
¼ cup salad oil
1 tablespoon lemon pepper
½ cup wine vinegar

½ cup Worcestershire sauce
¼ cup lemon juice
¼ cup soy sauce
½ teaspoon garlic salt

- Punch holes in roast with large kitchen fork and marinate overnight in mixture of next 7 ingredients, turning at least once.

- Drain marinade, leaving ½ cup in bottom of pan.

- Preheat oven to 450 degrees.

- Bake 5 minutes per pound, uncovered. Turn oven off, and leave in oven for 2½ hours. Remove immediately. Serves 8 to 10.

Alternate cooking method: Cook 1 hour per pound at 200 degrees for those who like their meat medium-well.

Dr. J. Roy Bourgoyne

Quick Pepper Steak

1½ pound flank steak, thinly sliced
2 tablespoons oil
1 envelope dry onion soup mix
1 (15-ounce) can Rotel tomatoes, chopped

1 green bell pepper, thinly sliced
1 teaspoon pepper
1 teaspoon soy sauce
1 teaspoon Worcestershire sauce
Cooked rice (optional)

- Brown meat strips in oil.

- Add all other ingredients and simmer 30 minutes. Serve over cooked rice. Serves 4.

Mrs. J. Howard McClain (Virginia)

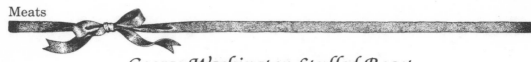

George Washington Stuffed Roast

4 or 5 pound sirloin tip roast
Tarragon vinegar
6 cloves garlic, peeled
Parsley
Celery tops
Green onion tops
¼ pound Parmesan cheese, cut in
small chunks

Suet
Salt and pepper to taste
⅛ teaspoon Tabasco
Flour, sifted
Dry Burgundy wine
Hot water

- Preheat oven to 350 degrees.

- Rub roast with tarragon vinegar and set aside.

- Chop individually, garlic, parsley, celery tops, green onion tops, Parmesan cheese, and a little suet.

- Keep each ingredient separate. Take paring knife and cut holes in roast 2 inches apart.

- Place a small amount of each ingredient in each hole.

- Sprinkle with salt and pepper.

- Add a few dashes Tabasco.

- Put a small amount of flour on top.

- Add ¼ cup dry Burgundy wine with every ½ cup hot water. (Use about 1 cup hot water when roast is put in oven.)

- Bake, covered, until medium done.

- Take out and refrigerate 24 hours.

- Put back in 350 degree oven, basting with more wine and hot water.

- Cook until done. Serves 10 to 12.

Mrs. Lyle E. Muller (Mary)

Bring roasts and steaks to room temperature before cooking.

For easier carving allow roast to stand 15 minutes after removing from oven.

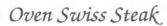

Oven Swiss Steak

1½ pound beef round steak,
  cut ¾-inch thick
¼ cup flour
1 teaspoon salt (optional)
2 tablespoons vegetable oil
1 (16-ounce) can stewed tomatoes
½ cup diced celery

½ cup diced carrot
2 tablespoons diced onion
½ teaspoon Worcestershire sauce
1 small can (individual serving) V-8
  Spicy Hot or Snappy Tom
¼ cup shredded sharp cheddar
  cheese (optional)

- Preheat oven to 350 degrees.

- Cut meat into 4 portions. Mix flour and salt, if used, and pound into meat. Set aside remaining flour.

- Brown meat in hot vegetable oil. Place meat in shallow baking dish.

- Blend flour with drippings in skillet. Add remaining ingredients except cheese. Cook, stirring constantly until mixture boils.

- Pour over meat. Cover. Bake 2 hours.

- Top with cheese if desired. Return to oven for few minutes. Serves 4.

Mrs. Ralph E. Knowles, Jr. (Janet)

Easy Five-Hour Beef Stew

3 pounds cubed stew meat
4 medium potatoes, quartered
3 onions, quartered
8 carrots, cut in large pieces
4 ribs celery, cut in large pieces
1 (28-ounce) can tomatoes
1 (10¾-ounce) can cream of
  mushroom soup

1 soup can water
1 envelope dry onion soup mix
1 tablespoon basil
4 tablespoons tapioca
Salt and pepper to taste

- Preheat oven to 275 degrees.

- Mix meat and vegetables in large roaster.

- Mash tomatoes and add soup, water, spices, and tapioca.

- Pour sauce over top and cover tightly. Bake 5 hours without opening oven! Serves 8 to 10.

Mrs. J. Roy Bourgoyne (Helen Ruth)

Beef Stew with Beer and Walnuts

3½ pounds lean boneless beef,
chuck or round
1 tablespoon Kitchen Bouquet
brown gravy seasoning
1 (12-ounce) can beer
1 envelope dry onion soup mix
1 (¾-ounce) envelope brown gravy
mix
1 teaspoon Worcestershire sauce

1 (10¾-ounce) can cream of
mushroom soup, undiluted
4 cups assorted frozen vegetables
(carrots, onions, broccoli, peas,
and cauliflower)
1 small loaf French bread per
serving
4 ounces walnut halves or pieces,
for garnish

- Trim away all fat from beef and cut into 1-inch cubes. Place in a 4-quart, ovenproof baking dish, or crockpot. Stir in Kitchen Bouquet to coat each slice of meat.

- Add beer, onion soup mix, brown gravy mix, and Worcestershire. Stir to blend. Cover dish tightly.

- Cook in oven at 200 to 225 degrees for 8 to 10 hours, or cook in crockpot on low for 10 hours. Stir in mushroom soup and frozen vegetables.

- Cook at same temperature 30 to 45 minutes until vegetables are tender.

- Serve in individual hollowed-out loaves of French bread or over rice. Top each with a sprinkle of walnuts. Makes 3 quarts of stew. Serves 6 to 8 people.

Mrs. Morris L. Robbins (Laura Dee)

Enchilada Casserole

1 pound ground beef
1 (15-ounce) can ranch style beans
6 frozen tortillas, thawed
1½ cups shredded cheddar cheese

1 (10-ounce) can Rotel tomatoes
1 (10¾-ounce) can cream of
mushroom soup

- Preheat oven to 350 degrees.

- Brown ground beef. Spread in greased 13x9x2-inch baking dish.

- Layer beans over beef. Top with tortillas and sprinkle with cheese. Spread tomatoes over tortillas and pour soup over all. Cover with aluminum foil and bake 1 hour. Serves 6.

Mrs. James E. Sexton (Pat)

Taco Casserole

2 pounds ground beef
1 medium onion, chopped
1 (8-ounce) can tomato sauce
1 (10-ounce) can enchilada sauce
Salt to taste

1 (12-ounce) package nacho flavor Doritos
8 ounces shredded sharp cheddar cheese

- Preheat oven to 350 degrees.

- Brown ground beef and onion on top of stove. Drain. Add tomato sauce, enchilada sauce, and salt.

- Line bottom and sides of 13x9x2-inch baking dish with Doritos and cover with meat filling. Top with cheese and bake 30 minutes. Serves 10 to 12.

Mrs. J. Roy Bourgoyne (Helen Ruth)

Company Meatloaf

1½ pounds ground chuck
¾ cup soft fine breadcrumbs
¼ cup ketchup
1 egg
1 teaspoon salt
3 to 4 pieces boiled ham, shaved
1 (10-ounce) package frozen chopped spinach, thawed and squeezed dry

¾ cup shredded mozzarella cheese
3 tablespoons freshly grated Parmesan cheese
¼ teaspoon thyme
½ teaspoon oregano
¼ teaspoon basil
¼ teaspoon garlic powder
3 tablespoons ketchup

- Combine ground chuck, breadcrumbs, ketchup, egg, and salt. Pat meat mixture on sheet of waxed paper 10x14-inches. Meat should be less than ½-inch thick.

- Place one layer of ham on top of meat.

- Combine spinach, cheeses, thyme, oregano, basil, and garlic powder. Spread mixture over ham, leaving ¾-inch margins. Roll as for jelly roll, pressing to seal edges.

- Chill in refrigerator 1 hour, time permitting.

- Preheat oven to 350 degrees.

- Place seam side down in broiler pan or on rack. Bake uncovered 1 hour. Spread ketchup on loaf and bake 15 more minutes. Serves 6.

Mrs. Michael J. Harty (Kay)

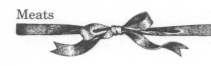

Moussaka

2 pounds ground chuck
2 medium onions, chopped
1 garlic clove, minced
4 tablespoons butter
1½ teaspoons salt
1 teaspoon pepper
¼ cup chopped parsley

1 (8-ounce) can tomato sauce
Dash nutmeg and cinnamon
1 cup water
3 eggs, beaten
3 large eggplants
1 cup grated Parmesan cheese

- Preheat oven to 350 degrees.

- Brown meat with onions, garlic, butter, salt, pepper, and parsley. Add tomato sauce, nutmeg, cinnamon, and water. Simmer 25 minutes.

- When cool, add eggs.

- Slice eggplants (do not peel) and soak in salt water for 15 minutes. Drain thoroughly. Fry in hot vegetable oil until brown. Drain on paper towels.

- Arrange alternate layers of cheese, eggplant, and meat mixture in an ungreased 13x9x2-inch baking dish.

Cream Sauce:
6 tablespoons butter, melted
5 tablespoons flour
3 cups milk
6 egg yolks, beaten

¼ cup grated Parmesan cheese
½ teaspoon salt
¼ teaspoon pepper

- Blend butter and flour together in heavy pan and slowly add 3 cups milk, stirring until thick. Add egg yolks, cheese, salt, and pepper. Pour sauce over eggplant and bake 45 minutes. Serves 8.

Mrs. J. Garland Cherry, Jr. (Carol)

Allow ¼ to ⅓ pound per serving when buying boneless meat; ⅓ to ½ pound meat with a bone; and ¾ to 1 pound for meat such as spareribs or shoulders.

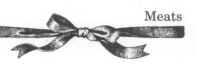

Manicotti

Cheese Filling:
1 pound ricotta cheese
12 ounces shredded mozzarella
cheese

2 whole eggs
½ cup grated Parmesan cheese

• Mix all ingredients for cheese filling and set aside.

Meat Sauce:
1 pound ground chuck
½ green bell pepper, chopped
1 onion, chopped
4 (16-ounce) cans tomato sauce

1 (6-ounce) can tomato paste
Salt, oregano, and garlic powder
to taste

• Brown meat; add pepper and onion. Mix well. Add tomato sauce, tomato paste, salt, oregano, and garlic powder. Cook for 2 hours.

1 (10-ounce) box manicotti noodles

• Preheat oven to 350 degrees.

• Cook noodles according to directions on box. Cool slightly. Fill noodles with cheese mixture.

• Pour half of sauce into 13x9x2-inch baking dish. Place filled manicotti noodles over sauce. Pour remaining sauce over noodles. Cover with aluminum foil. Bake 45 minutes. Serves 12.

Mrs. Hilbert Nease (Betty)

If pasta is cooked in advance, drain and toss with oil. Refrigerate covered with a damp cloth. Before serving, dip in boiling water for 2 seconds.

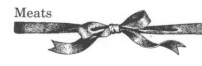

Lasagna Casserole

1 pound hot sausage
1 pound ground beef
1 clove garlic
1 teaspoon whole basil
1 teaspoon oregano
1 teaspoon salt
1 (16-ounce) can tomatoes
2 (6-ounce) cans tomato paste
1 (10-ounce) box lasagna

4 cups creamy small curd cottage
  cheese
¾ cup grated Parmesan cheese
2 tablespoons parsley flakes
3 eggs, beaten
½ teaspoon salt
½ teaspoon pepper
16 ounces sliced mozzarella cheese

- Brown sausage and ground beef in skillet.

- Add next 6 ingredients for meat sauce. Simmer uncovered 30 minutes. Set aside.

- Cook lasagna noodles according to package and drain.

- Combine cottage cheese, Parmesan cheese, parsley, eggs, salt, and pepper.

- Preheat oven to 350 degrees.

- Place layer of cooked noodles in greased 13x9x2-inch baking dish. Spread with half of cheese mixture. Top with half of mozzarella cheese and cover with half of meat sauce.

- Repeat layers, topping with remaining mozzarella cheese slices. Bake 30 minutes. Cool 10 minutes before cutting into squares. Serves 10.

Mrs. J. Garland Cherry, Jr. (Carol)
Mrs. Richard C. Harris (Beverly)

When cooking dried pasta, add a small amount of vegetable oil to water to reduce splashing and prevent sticking. Add pasta all at once to boiling water.

Stuffed Pasta Shells

18 jumbo shells (#95)
1 pound ground chuck
1 large onion, chopped
1 clove garlic, chopped
8 ounces shredded mozzarella
  cheese
½ cup breadcrumbs

¼ cup chopped parsley
1 egg
Salt and pepper to taste
2 (15½-ounce) jars spaghetti sauce
⅓ cup dry wine
½ cup grated Parmesan cheese

- Preheat oven to 400 degrees.

- Cook shells about 15 minutes. Drain and set aside.

- In skillet brown ground meat, onion, and garlic until crumbly. Drain excess fat and cool.

- Stir in mozzarella, breadcrumbs, parsley, egg, salt, and pepper. Mix well and stuff shells.

- Spoon half of sauce into 13x9x2-inch baking dish and place shells on top of sauce in a single layer.

- Mix wine with remaining sauce and pour over shells. Sprinkle with Parmesan cheese. Bake 20 to 25 minutes or until brown and bubbly. Serves 8 to 10.

Mrs. James R. Ross (Lucy)

Tamale Casserole

1 (15-ounce) can chili (without
  beans)
1 (14-ounce) can tamales
1 (10-ounce) package frozen corn

1 (6-ounce) can ripe olives
1 cup shredded sharp cheddar
  cheese
1½ cups corn chips, crushed

- Preheat oven to 350 degrees.

- Spread a layer of chili on bottom of 8x8x2-inch greased casserole.

- Cut tamales in bite size pieces and spread over chili. Layer corn on top of tamales. Layer ripe olives on top of corn. Repeat until tamales, corn, and olives are used. Spread cheese on top and cover with crushed corn chips.

- Bake 30 minutes until bubbly. Serves 6.

Mrs. Chester Lloyd (Betty)

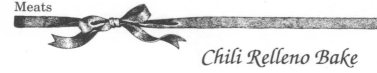

Chili Relleno Bake

½ **pound each, bulk pork sausage and lean ground beef**
1 large onion, chopped
1 clove garlic, minced or pressed
2 (4-ounce) cans whole California green chilies, drained and seeded
2 cups shredded sharp cheddar cheese

4 eggs
¼ **cup flour**
1½ **cups milk**
1 teaspoon salt
⅛ **to** ¼ **teaspoon liquid hot pepper seasoning**

- Preheat oven to 350 degrees.

- Crumble sausage and beef in skillet on medium heat. Stir until brown; drain. Add onion and garlic and cook until onion is limp. Set aside.

- Line an 8-inch square baking dish with half the chilies. Top with 1½ cups cheese, meat mixture, and remaining chilies.

- Beat eggs and flour together until smooth. Add milk, salt, and hot pepper seasoning, beating well. Pour over meat mixture and sprinkle with remaining cheese.

- Bake 45 minutes or until knife inserted in center comes out clean. Let stand 5 minutes. Serves 6.

Mrs. James W. Clark (Carolyn)

Country Ham

12 to 18 pound Tennessee country ham

Water to cover

- Scrub ham thoroughly with stiff brush to remove mold.

- Place in roaster or other container with tight fitting lid. Cover completely with water and bring to a full rolling boil without lid.

- Cover and remove to out-of-the-way place. Completely wrap container in newspaper and old blankets to hold in heat.

- Allow to set a full twenty-four hours. Remove from container, trim fat and brown quickly under broiler. Slice thinly and serve hot or cold.

Mrs. John Mallett Barron (Doy)

Apricot Stuffed Pork

1 (12-ounce) package dried apricots
1 cup boiling water
4½ to 5 pound pork loin center rib roast
¼ teaspoon pepper

¼ teaspoon salt
½ teaspoon ground ginger
4 tablespoons red currant jelly (or apricot jelly)

- Soak apricots in boiling water for 30 minutes. Drain and pat dry.

- Preheat oven to 325 degrees.

- With long narrow sharp knife, pierce through center of roast from one end to the other, twisting slit in the meat (or have butcher prepare meat).

- Stuff apricots into slit.

- Season roast with pepper, salt, and ginger.

- Place roast in shallow open roasting pan; insert meat thermometer being careful not to touch bone or stuffing.

- Bake 2 to 2½ hours or until thermometer reads 170 degrees F.

- Melt jelly over low heat and spread over roast that has been placed on platter. Serves 8 to 10.

The red currant jelly forms a beautiful glaze.
The handle of a wooden spoon is a good tool to use to stuff roast.

Mrs. Lyle E. Muller (Mary)

Pork Chops Supreme

6 loin pork chops, cut 1-inch thick
6 slices onion
6 slices lemon

6 tablespoons brown sugar
6 tablespoons ketchup

- Preheat oven to 350 degrees.

- Place chops in shallow baking dish.

- Place one slice onion and lemon on each chop. Put 1 tablespoon brown sugar and ketchup on top of each chop.

- Cover dish tightly and bake 1 hour. Uncover, baste with drippings and bake an additional 30 minutes. Serves 6.

Mrs. Joe Hall Morris (Adair)

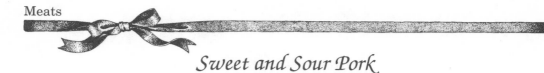

Sweet and Sour Pork

6 medium pork chops
2 eggs, beaten
Cornstarch
Vegetable oil
1 carrot, sliced
2 tablespoons vegetable oil
1 green bell pepper, cored and
  sliced
1 small onion, sliced

1 (14-ounce) can pineapple chunks
Water
2 tablespoons soy sauce
½ cup wine vinegar
¼ cup brown sugar
½ teaspoon garlic powder
½ cup cornstarch
½ cup water
Cooked noodles or rice (optional)

- Cut meat from bone, removing fat. Cut meat into 1-inch cubes. Dip into beaten egg and roll in cornstarch.

- Pour enough oil in skillet to make 2-inch depth.

- Fry pork cubes in hot oil about 5 minutes until crisp.

- Parboil carrots.

- Heat 2 tablespoons oil in skillet.

- Stir-fry green bell pepper and onion 2 minutes.

- Drain pineapple, adding enough water to juice to make 1 cup.

- Combine pineapple, juice, soy sauce, vinegar, brown sugar, garlic powder, browned pork, and carrots in skillet. Heat to boiling.

- Blend cornstarch with water until smooth and add to skillet.

- Cook over medium heat until bubbly and clear.

- Serve over crisp noodles or fluffy hot rice. Makes 6 servings.

Mrs. Thomas E. Gulledge (Mildred)

Before opening a package of bacon, roll it into a tube. The slices will be easier to separate.

Pork Tenderloin

½ to 1 pound pork tenderloin
Vegetable oil
Salt, pepper, granulated garlic, and
  oregano to taste

Juice of 1 lemon

- Preheat oven to 350 degrees.

- Bring meat to room temperature and coat with vegetable oil. Rub generously with salt, pepper, and granulated garlic. Sprinkle lightly with oregano.

- Bake about 45 minutes. Remove from oven and sprinkle with lemon juice. Serves 2 to 3.

Mrs. James G. Sousoulas (Sophie)

Ham Roll Ups

2 (10½-ounce) cans cream of mushroom soup
1 pint sour cream
2 cups cottage cheese
2 eggs, beaten
½ cup finely chopped green onion

1 (10-ounce) package frozen
  chopped spinach, cooked and
  drained well
1 teaspoon dry mustard
½ teaspoon salt
30 slices thinly sliced cooked ham

- Combine soup and ½ cup sour cream and set aside for sauce.

- Combine rest of sour cream, cottage cheese, eggs, onion, spinach, mustard, and salt. Mix well and chill several hours.

- Preheat oven to 350 degrees.

- Spoon approximately 1 tablespoon filling on each ham slice and roll up.

- Place close together, seam side down, in 13x9x2-inch baking dish.

- Spoon sauce over all.

- Bake 20 to 25 minutes until bubbly. Serves 6.

Mrs. Thomas R. Meadows (Karen)

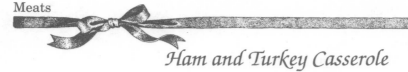

Ham and Turkey Casserole

½ cup margarine
¼ cup flour
2 cups milk
1 (6-ounce) can mushrooms
2 teaspoons instant onion
2 teaspoons prepared mustard
1 cup sour cream
5 ounces cooked noodles
  (about 2 cups)

1½ cups cubed ham
1½ cups cubed turkey
1 (8-ounce) can sliced water
  chestnuts
1 (2-ounce) jar chopped pimentos
Slivered almonds

- Preheat oven to 325 degrees.
- Melt margarine. Add flour and slowly add milk, stirring constantly.
- Cook until thick and bubbly; set aside.
- Mix next 9 ingredients and combine with above sauce.
- Pour into 2-quart casserole.
- Sprinkle with slivered almonds.
- Bake 30 minutes. Serves 6 to 8.

Great for leftover ham and turkey after the holidays.

Mrs. Frank J. Hudson (Bettye)

Use Coca-Cola to baste a ham.

Ham and Vegetable Casserole

4 (10-ounce) packages frozen mixed
  vegetables
3 cups fresh bread cubes
½ cup butter or margarine, melted
1 cup flour
1 teaspoon salt
¼ teaspoon pepper
2 teaspoons dry mustard

2 teaspoons Worcestershire sauce
5 cups milk
¾ cup butter or margarine
1 medium onion, grated
8 ounces sharp cheddar cheese,
  shredded
2 pounds cooked ham, cubed

- Preheat oven to 350 degrees when ready to bake.

- Cook vegetables as directed on package. Do not overcook. Set aside.

- Toss bread cubes in melted butter and refrigerate.

- Mix next 5 ingredients, add milk slowly, add butter and cook until thickened,
  stirring constantly. Add onion, cheese, ham, and drained vegetables. Pour into two
  11x7x2-inch greased baking dishes.

- Refrigerate overnight. Top with bread cubes and bake 30 to 45 minutes. Serves 25.

Mrs. J. Roy Bourgoyne (Helen Ruth)

Roast Leg of Lamb

1 4 to 6 pound leg of lamb
½ cup lemon juice
¼ cup olive oil
1 large clove garlic, crushed
½ teaspoon coarsely ground pepper

½ teaspoon thyme
½ teaspoon basil
½ teaspoon lemon pepper
½ teaspoon salt

- Preheat oven to 325 degrees.

- Place leg of lamb in shallow pan.

- Mix lemon juice, olive oil, garlic, and seasonings; pour over meat. Turn roast until
  well coated. Roast 25 to 30 minutes per pound. Reserve marinade for gravy.

Cookbook Committee

Lamb Shanks Milanaise

4 lamb shanks
¼ cup plus 2 tablespoons flour
¼ teaspoon pepper
¼ cup plus 2 tablespoons vegetable
 oil

1 cup white wine
¼ cup chicken bouillon
1 clove garlic, minced
1 tablespoon dried parsley
1 tablespoon lemon juice

- Trim excess fat from lamb; rinse and pat dry. Combine flour and pepper; dredge lamb.

- Heat oil in skillet, add lamb, and cook over medium heat until browned. Drain oil from skillet; add wine to lamb and cook 5 minutes. Reduce heat and add bouillon and seasonings. Cover and simmer 4 hours until lamb is tender. You may bake in 325 degree oven 4 hours. If mixture becomes too dry or thick, add more bouillon. Serves 4.

Mrs. Cecil L. Raines (Ann)

Veal Scallops in White Wine Sauce

5 thin veal scallops, seasoned with
 salt and pepper
½ cup butter
1½ pounds mushrooms, thinly
 sliced

¼ cup Calvados or cognac
½ cup white wine
4 tablespoons heavy cream

- Heat 3 tablespoons butter in saucepan and add veal. Cook over low heat without browning, turning only once.

- Remove veal and place it with slices overlapping on a service platter. Cover and keep warm.

- Reduce the liquid until it is almost syrup. Add 1½ tablespoons butter and the mushrooms. Cook over high heat until liquid is almost evaporated.

- Add the Calvados or cognac, and white wine, cook until reduced by half.

- Add the cream, cooking over medium heat until thickened. Remove from heat and stir in remaining butter.

- Pour over veal slices. Serves 5.

Dr. Richard J. Reynolds

Grilled Catfish with Dijon Sauce

4 catfish fillets
3 tablespoons butter or margarine, melted

1 teaspoon Worcestershire sauce
1 teaspoon lemon pepper

- Rinse fillets and blot dry.

- Combine butter, Worcestershire, and lemon pepper. Mix well. Brush both sides of fillets with butter mixture and place on sheet of heavy foil or in well-greased fish basket.

- Grill over medium hot coals 5 minutes. Turn fillets and grill 5 minutes or until fish flakes easily when tested with a fork.

- For oven cooking, broil fish 6 inches from heat 10 to 12 minutes.

Dijon Sauce:
½ cup sour cream
1 tablespoon Dijon mustard

1 teaspoon Worcestershire sauce
Lemon twists (optional)

- Combine ingredients.

- Heat 45 seconds in microwave or until warm. Serve 2 tablespoons sauce over each catfish fillet and garnish with lemon.

Dr. Phillip Sherman, Jr.

Parmesan Catfish Fillets

4 catfish fillets
1 egg
1 tablespoon milk
1 cup grated Parmesan cheese

¼ cup flour
Dash cayenne
Salt to taste

- Preheat oven to 350 degrees.

- Beat egg and milk together.

- Dip catfish into liquid mixture, then dip in dry mixture made up of cheese, flour, cayenne, and salt. Coat well on all sides.

- Bake uncovered in greased 11x7x2-inch baking dish 30 minutes. Serves 4.

Mrs. Phillip Sherman, Sr. (Barbara)

Crabmeat Supreme in Coquille

¼ cup margarine
2 tablespoons flour
1 teaspoon prepared mustard
½ teaspoon horseradish
Dash pepper
¾ teaspoon salt

1 teaspoon onion juice
1 cup milk
2 hard-boiled eggs, chopped
1 pound crabmeat
½ cup cracker crumbs

- Preheat oven to 400 degrees.

- Melt margarine, blend in flour, and bring to boil. Boil for 1 minute. Add mustard, horseradish, pepper, salt, onion juice, and milk. Bring to boil and cook until thickened, stirring constantly. Add chopped eggs and crabmeat. Stir and mix well.

- Place in 11x7x2-inch baking dish, dot with butter, and top with cracker crumbs. Bake 15 minutes. Serves 6.

Crabmeat mixture may be served in pastry shells. Sprinkle with paprika.

Mrs. James L. Wiygul (Lou)

Deviled Crab

1 cup milk
2 tablespoons butter or margarine, softened
2 tablespoons flour
2 eggs, beaten
2 tablespoons mayonnaise
2 teaspoons Worcestershire sauce
1 teaspoon Dijon mustard
1½ teaspoons salt
¼ teaspoon red pepper

Juice of 1 lemon
2 tablespoons sherry
½ bottle capers (optional)
1 pound crabmeat
½ pound shrimp, cooked and deveined
2 tablespoons butter or margarine, melted
⅔ cup soft breadcrumbs

- Preheat oven to 325 degrees.

- Scald milk in double boiler.

- Blend butter and flour; add eggs, mayonnaise, Worcestershire, mustard, salt and pepper. Stir into scalded milk and cook until thick, stirring constantly. Add lemon juice, sherry, capers, crab, and shrimp.

- Pour into 2-quart casserole or 6 individual ramekins. Combine melted butter with breadcrumbs and sprinkle over top. Bake 20 to 30 minutes. Serves 6.

Mrs. P. D. Miller, Jr. (Greene)

Eggplant Supreme with Crabmeat

1 medium eggplant
Boiling salted water
2 tablespoons butter
¼ cup finely chopped onion
⅓ cup finely chopped celery
¼ cup finely chopped green bell
   pepper

1 teaspoon salt
½ teaspoon pepper
½ teaspoon curry powder
1 (6½-ounce) can lump or flaked
   crabmeat, drained
Grated Parmesan cheese

- Preheat oven to 350 degrees.

- Cut eggplant in quarters. Scoop out and reserve pulp, leaving about ⅜-inch shell.

- Cook shells in boiling salted water for 4 minutes and drain.

- Sauté onion, celery, and green bell pepper in butter until glazed. Add chopped pulp, salt, pepper, and curry powder. Cook until eggplant is done. Add crabmeat and cook 2 minutes.

- Fill shells with mixture. Sprinkle with Parmesan cheese and place in lightly buttered shallow pan. Bake 30 minutes. Serves 4.

Mrs. G. W. Huckaba (Ann)

Creole Style Halibut

2 tablespoons margarine
1 tablespoon flour
1 tablespoon minced green bell
   pepper
1 tablespoon minced onion

2 cups cooked tomatoes
⅛ teaspoon salt
⅛ teaspoon pepper
2 pounds halibut steaks

- Preheat oven to 400 degrees.

- Melt margarine and blend in flour. Add green pepper and onion. Cook 3 minutes. Add tomatoes and cook until thickened, stirring constantly. Simmer 10 minutes longer.

- Rub mixture through strainer and season with salt and pepper.

- Place halibut steaks in lightly greased 13x9x2-inch baking dish. Pour Creole sauce over fish. Bake 30 minutes. Serves 4.

May substitute red snapper for halibut.

Mrs. James L. Wiygul (Lou)

Poached Salmon with Dilled Hollandaise Sauce

1 quart water
1 cup dry white wine
1 small onion, sliced
1 small carrot
1 teaspoon salt
3 or 4 peppercorns

1 bay leaf
Parsley sprig
1 rib celery
Pinch thyme
2 to 3 pounds salmon fillets

- Put 1 quart of water in a fish kettle and add all ingredients except salmon fillets. Bring to a boil and simmer 20 minutes.

- Wrap salmon fillets in cheese cloth, lower onto rack in kettle, and simmer gently about 20 minutes. Make sauce while fillets are cooking.

Sauce:
3 egg yolks
½ cup plus 2 tablespoons butter,
　softened

2 teaspoons lemon juice
⅛ teaspoon salt
½ teaspoon dried dill weed

- Mix egg yolks in a small, heavy saucepan.

- Stir in softened butter, a tablespoon at a time, over low heat. Add second table-spoon of butter when first has melted, until all butter is incorporated. Stir in lemon juice, salt and dill weed. Stir constantly. Be patient, it will thicken if fire is low.

Garnish:
Lemon slices
Parsley

Watercress
Cucumber

- Remove fish from liquid, unwrap and carefully remove skin.

- Arrange salmon on a hot platter. Garnish with lemon slice, parsley, watercress, and cucumber. Serve with sauce. Serves 6 to 8.

Mrs. Richard J. Reynolds (Anne)

To freeze fish, place in pan of water or other container and freeze so that it is encased in a block of ice. Remove from pan and wrap well. This can be kept for 2 months.

Baked Salmon Steaks

4 salmon steaks, cut 1 inch thick
⅓ cup margarine, melted
1 teaspoon Worcestershire sauce

1 teaspoon grated onion
¼ teaspoon paprika

• Preheat oven to 350 degrees.

• Place steaks in an 11x7x2-inch baking dish.

• Blend ingredients and brush lightly on the steaks, saving the remaining sauce to serve during the meal.

• Sprinkle lightly with salt. Bake 25 to 30 minutes. Serves 4.

Mrs. James L. Wiygul (Lou)

Seafood Casserole Royale

2 (10½-ounce) cans condensed
  cream of shrimp soup
½ cup mayonnaise
1 small onion, grated
¾ cup milk
Salt, white pepper, seasoned salt,
  ground nutmeg and cayenne to
  taste
3 pounds cooked shrimp
1 (7½-ounce) can crabmeat, drained

1 (6-ounce) can water chestnuts,
  drained and sliced
1½ cups diced celery
3 tablespoons fresh parsley, minced
1⅓ cups white long-grain rice,
  cooked until dry and fluffy
Paprika
1 (2-ounce) package slivered
  almonds

• Preheat oven to 350 degrees.

• Blend soup and mayonnaise in a large bowl. Stir until smooth. Add onion, then milk. Add rest of ingredients except paprika and almonds.

• Check seasonings, adding more to taste. If mixture seems dry add a few table-spoons of milk to moisten.

• Sprinkle almonds and paprika over top. Bake uncovered in 13x9x2-inch baking dish 30 minutes, or until hot and bubbly. Serves 10.

Freezes well.

Mrs. George H. Bouldien (Judy)

Seafood and Wild Rice Casserole

2 tablespoons butter
1½ cups chopped celery
1½ cups chopped onion
1 green bell pepper, chopped
1½ pounds cooked seafood (shrimp, crab, etc.)
1 (6-ounce) package wild and long grain rice, cooked

1 (4-ounce) jar mushrooms and juice
1 (4-ounce) jar pimentos and juice
2 (10¾-ounce) cans cream of mushroom soup, undiluted
2 tablespoons cooking sherry
½ cup breadcrumbs

• Preheat oven to 350 degrees.

• Sauté celery, onion, and pepper in butter. Add next 6 ingredients and mix well.

• Put into greased 13x9x2-inch baking dish. Top with breadcrumbs. Bake 30 minutes or until hot. Serves 8.

Mrs. Richard J. Reynolds (Anne)

Shrimp Creole

½ pound bacon, diced
3 green bell peppers, chopped
4 onions, chopped
2 cloves garlic, finely chopped
4 cups chopped celery
½ cup chopped parsley
3 (28-ounce) cans tomatoes

½ teaspoon pepper
1 teaspoon salt
1 teaspoon curry powder
1 teaspoon thyme
½ teaspoon cayenne
5 pounds raw shrimp, cleaned
Cooked rice

• Sauté peppers, onions, garlic, celery, and parsley with bacon pieces.

• Add tomatoes and seasonings and cook slowly 30 minutes.

• Add shrimp and cook 20 minutes. Serve over rice. Serves 8 to 10.

Mrs. Phillip Sherman, Jr. (Sandy)

Shrimp Creole and Rice

6 to 8 slices bacon
3 tablespoons margarine
1 large onion, chopped
1 clove garlic, crushed
2 cups chopped celery
8 ounces mushrooms, sliced
1 (28-ounce) can whole tomatoes
4 tablespoons tomato paste
3 cups chicken broth

½ teaspoon thyme
¼ teaspoon red pepper
¼ teaspoon paprika
1 teaspoon salt
1½ cups sliced okra
¼ cup chopped parsley
5 pounds shrimp, cooked, shelled
  and deveined

- Fry and crumble bacon. Set aside.

- Melt margarine; sauté onion, garlic, celery, and mushrooms. Put in Dutch oven. Add bacon, tomatoes, tomato paste, broth, spices, and okra. Simmer 1 hour. Add parsley and shrimp; simmer 15 minutes. Serve over rice.

Rice:
2 cups uncooked rice
2 (10¾-ounce) cans French onion
  soup

2 (10¾-ounce) cans water
2 teaspoons salt
½ cup butter, melted

- Preheat oven to 350 degrees.

- Mix all ingredients. Pour into 13x9x2-inch baking dish. Bake covered 1 hour, stirring once. Serves 8.

Mrs. P. D. Miller, Jr. (Greene)

Shrimp in Lemon Butter

1 cup butter
¼ cup lemon juice
1 clove garlic, minced
1 teaspoon parsley flakes
1 teaspoon Worcestershire sauce
1 teaspoon soy sauce
½ teaspoon coarsely ground black
  pepper

¼ teaspoon salt
¼ teaspoon garlic salt
2 pounds large shrimp, peeled and
  deveined
Lemon wedges (optional)

- Melt butter in large skillet. Add next 8 ingredients and bring to boil. Add shrimp; cook over medium heat 5 minutes, stirring occasionally. Garnish shrimp with lemon wedges if desired. Serves 4 to 6.

Mrs. George H. Bouldien (Judy)

Parmesan Shrimp au Gratin with Sherry

4 cups water
1 tablespoon salt

1½ pounds shrimp

- Heat water and salt to boiling. Add shrimp and simmer 1 to 3 minutes until shrimp turn pink. Drain and rinse in cold water to stop cooking process; rinse and drain again.

Cheese Sauce:
2 tablespoons butter or margarine
2 tablespoons flour
¼ teaspoon salt
Dash pepper
1 tablespoon parsley flakes
1 tablespoon Louisiana hot sauce (optional)

1¼ cups milk
2 cups shredded cheddar cheese
1 tablespoon lemon juice
1 tablespoon Worcestershire sauce
2 tablespoons sherry

- Melt butter. Stir in flour, salt, pepper, parsley, and hot sauce; add milk all at once. Cook over medium heat, stirring until thickened and bubbly.

- Add cheese and stir until melted. Add lemon juice, Worcestershire, and sherry; cook 1 minute.

- Arrange shrimp in 11x7x2-inch baking dish. Pour sauce over shrimp.

Topping:
½ cup shredded cheddar cheese

¼ cup grated Parmesan cheese

- Sprinkle cheddar cheese over sauce in dish and top with Parmesan cheese. Broil until cheese melts. Serves 4 to 6.

Good with rice, pasta, or baked potato and salad.

Mrs. William K. Barrett, III (Wanza)

*T*o remove the odor of shrimp while cooking, drop fresh celery leaves in the pot.

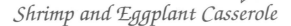

Shrimp and Eggplant Casserole

3 large eggplants
Salted water
1 pound frozen shrimp, peeled and
  deveined
1 bunch scallions, chopped
1 (4-ounce) can button mushrooms
3 tablespoons butter
¼ pound crackers, crushed

1 (10¾-ounce) can cream of
  mushroom soup
¼ cup dry sherry
Salt and pepper to taste
Dash Tabasco
¾ cup shredded mild cheddar
  cheese

- Peel and cube eggplant. Boil until soft in salted water. Add shrimp and cook 15 to 20 more minutes.

- As shrimp cook, sauté scallions and mushrooms in butter until soft.

- Drain liquid from cooked eggplant and shrimp; use to moisten crackers.

- Preheat oven to 350 degrees.

- Combine all ingredients, except cheese, and put into 13x9x2-inch casserole. Top with cheese. Bake covered 1 hour.

- Remove cover and cook a little longer if casserole is too moist. Serves 6.

Can be baked in eggplant shells.

Mrs. William H. McHorris (Jackie)

Two pounds of unpeeled shrimp properly cooked, will yield one pound cooked, peeled, deveined shrimp.

Shrimp, Mushroom and Artichoke Casserole

2½ tablespoons butter
8 ounces fresh mushrooms
1 (20-ounce) can artichoke hearts
1½ pounds cooked shrimp
4½ tablespoons butter
4½ tablespoons flour
¾ cup milk

¾ cup whipping cream
½ cup dry cooking sherry
1 tablespoon Worcestershire sauce
Salt and pepper to taste
½ cup grated Parmesan cheese
Paprika
Cooked rice

- Preheat oven to 375 degrees.

- Melt 2½ tablespoons butter and sauté mushrooms; set aside.

- In 2-quart casserole, layer artichoke hearts, shrimp, and mushrooms.

- Make sauce by melting 4½ tablespoons butter; add flour, stirring with whisk. Add milk and cream; stir until thick. Add sherry, Worcestershire, salt, and pepper to cream sauce. Pour sauce over layered ingredients.

- Top with Parmesan cheese and sprinkle with paprika. Bake 20 to 30 minutes. Serve over rice. Serves 6.

Mrs. Dan T. Meadows (Amy)

Southwest Shrimp Casserole

1 (4-ounce) jar mushrooms and
    pieces
¼ pound margarine, melted
1 pound cooked shrimp
2 cups cooked rice
½ cup chopped green bell pepper

½ cup chopped onion
½ cup chopped celery
2½ cups canned tomatoes, drained
¾ teaspoon salt
1 tablespoon chili powder

- Preheat oven to 300 degrees.

- Combine all ingredients and place in greased 13x9x2-inch baking dish. Bake 1 hour. If mixture gets dry while cooking, add juice drained from tomatoes. Serves 6.

Mrs. Frank J. Hudson (Bettye)

Shrimp Victoria

1 small onion, chopped
¾ pound shrimp, peeled and
   deveined
2 tablespoons butter
2½ ounces mushrooms

1½ teaspoons flour
½ teaspoon salt
½ cup sour cream
Cooking sherry to taste
Cooked rice

- Sauté onion and shrimp in butter for 10 minutes. Add mushrooms and sauté 5 more minutes. Sprinkle in flour and salt. Keep on low heat and add sour cream. Cook 10 more minutes. Add sherry.

- Serve over rice.

Mrs. Stephen Weir (Dottie)

Company Tuna

¼ cup butter
¼ cup margarine
1 cup sliced fresh mushrooms
1 cup diced celery
¾ cup coarsely chopped frozen
   green bell pepper
4 tablespoons flour
2½ cups milk
2 tablespoons dried onion
½ teaspoon paprika

2 teaspoons seasoned salt
1 teaspoon salt
¼ teaspoon pepper
3 (6½-ounce) cans albacore tuna,
   packed in water
½ cup pimento strips, finely
   chopped
3 tablespoons dry sherry
Sliced almonds

- Melt butter and margarine. Sauté mushrooms, celery, and bell pepper. When tender, lower heat and stir in flour.

- Cook a few minutes, stirring frequently, and slowly add milk. Add dried onion, paprika, seasoned salt, salt, and pepper. Bring to boil and stir occasionally. Add tuna and drained pimento.

- Immediately before serving, add 3 tablespoons dry sherry. Serve in patty shells. Garnish with sliced almonds. Yields 6 cups.

Mrs. Joe Hall Morris (Adair)

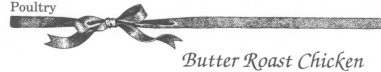

Butter Roast Chicken

8 chicken breast halves, boned and
  skinned
¼ pound butter or margarine
Juice of 2 lemons
2 teaspoons salt
1 teaspoon pepper

3 teaspoons paprika
½ teaspoon brown sugar
Dash Tabasco
⅛ teaspoon powdered rosemary
⅛ teaspoon nutmeg

• Preheat oven to 325 degrees.

• Wash chicken in cold water and pat dry.

• Melt butter and add remaining ingredients to make sauce. Stir well over low heat
  until seasonings are well blended.

• Using pastry brush, brush sauce over chicken. Place on rack in shallow pan and
  roast approximately 2 hours, basting with sauce every 12 to 15 minutes. Serves 8.

Dr. Joe Hall Morris

Chicken a la Crème

White Sauce:
8 tablespoons butter
8 tablespoons flour

1 teaspoon salt
4 cups milk

• Melt butter. Stir in flour and salt. Add milk and cook over low heat until thickened.

6 cups chopped cooked chicken
2 cups sliced mushrooms, fresh or
  canned
1 (4-ounce) jar chopped pimento
1 teaspoon onion juice

⅛ teaspoon salt
⅛ teaspoon cayenne
Sherry to taste
4 egg yolks

• Combine all ingredients except egg yolks. Heat thoroughly.

• Add egg yolks right before serving while chicken and cream sauce are still warm.
  Makes 8 dinner servings.

Great served in miniature patty shells for teas, luncheons, or cocktail buffets.

Mrs. Phillip Sherman, Jr. (Sandy)

Chicken Breasts Supreme

1 (2½-ounce) jar dried beef
8 slices bacon
4 chicken breasts, skinned, halved and boned
2 cups sour cream
1 (10¾-ounce) can cream of mushroom soup

1 (3-ounce) package cream cheese, softened
Cooked rice
Paprika

- Preheat oven to 325 degrees.

- In buttered 13x9x2-inch baking dish, place beef slices.

- Wrap one slice of bacon around each breast half and place in casserole.

- Mix sour cream, soup, and cream cheese and pour over chicken. Cover and bake 2½ hours. Bake uncovered the last 30 minutes.

- Serve over rice. Sprinkle with paprika. Serves 4.

Especially good for summer buffet.

Mrs. O'Farrell Shoemaker (Melanie)

Chicken and Rice Delight

4 cups cooked and diced chicken
2 teaspoons lemon juice
1 cup cooked rice
1 (2-ounce) jar pimentos, drained
1 teaspoon minced onion
¾ cup mayonnaise
1 cup chopped celery
4 hard-boiled eggs

1 (10¾-ounce) can cream of chicken soup
1 (10¾-ounce) can cream of mushroom soup
Garlic salt to taste
Salt and pepper to taste
1 cup shredded cheddar cheese
1½ cups crumbled potato chips

- Mix all ingredients except cheese and chips. Pour into 13x9x2-inch baking dish. Place in refrigerator overnight.

- Preheat oven to 400 degrees.

- Top with cheese and potato chips and bake for 25 minutes. Serves 6 to 8.

Mrs. Weber W. Manning (Robin)

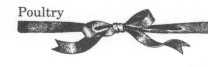

Chicken Marsala

6 chicken breast halves, skinned and boned
½ cup flour combined with salt, white pepper, and paprika to taste
1 cup margarine, melted
1 pound fresh mushrooms, quartered

1 (13¾-ounce) can chicken broth
½ cup Marsala wine
1 (8-ounce) package sliced mozzarella cheese
½ cup grated Parmesan cheese

- Preheat oven to 350 degrees.

- Flatten chicken breasts between two pieces of waxed paper using mallet or rolling pin. Lightly dust chicken with flour mixture and sauté in melted margarine until golden brown.

- Transfer chicken to 11x7x2-inch baking dish, reserving margarine and chicken drippings in skillet to sauté mushrooms. Transfer mushrooms to casserole, leaving drippings in skillet, and adding chicken broth and wine. Simmer 15 to 20 minutes.

- Layer cheeses on top of chicken breasts and pour wine sauce in casserole. Bake 30 minutes. Serves 6.

Mrs. Justin D. Towner (Ginny)

Chicken Enchilada Casserole

1 (3-pound) chicken
1 (10¾-ounce) can cream of mushroom soup
1 (10¾-ounce) can cream of chicken soup
1 cup chicken broth
1 (4-ounce) can chopped green chilies

1 teaspoon chili powder
⅛ teaspoon garlic powder
¼ teaspoon pepper
4 teaspoons minced onion
4 cups corn chips or tortilla chips
1 (8-ounce) package shredded sharp cheddar cheese
½ cup fried onion rings

- Cook and bone chicken and cut into small pieces. Reserve 1 cup broth.

- Preheat oven to 350 degrees.

- Combine soups, broth, green chilies, and all spices. Blend well.

- Cover bottom of 13x9x2-inch baking dish with chips. Alternate layers of chicken, soup mixture, cheese, and chips, ending with cheese.

- Sprinkle top with crushed onion rings. Bake 50 minutes. Serves 8.

Mrs. C. Dale Moody, Jr. (Doris)

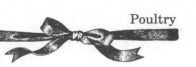

Chicken Crescents

3 (10-ounce) tubes crescent dinner rolls

2 (1-ounce) packages McCormick gravy mix

Filling:
1 (3-ounce) package cream cheese
4 teaspoons grated onion
6 tablespoons soft margarine
6 teaspoons lemon pepper

3 cups cooked chicken, finely chopped
1 (4-ounce) jar chopped mushrooms

- Combine cream cheese, onion, margarine, and lemon pepper. Add chicken and mushrooms. Set aside.

Coating Mix:
1 cup herb-stuffing mix
¾ cup chopped pecans

¾ cup margarine, melted

- Combine coating mix ingredients and set aside.

- Preheat oven to 375 degrees.

- Separate rolls into triangular sections. Place 2 tablespoons of filling in the center of each roll. Fold according to directions, tucking in edges and corners.

- Roll crescents in coating mix and place on foil-lined 15x10x1-inch baking sheet. Bake 20 minutes or until golden brown.

- Prepare gravy mix according to package directions. Spoon gravy over crescents when ready to serve. Serves 8 to 10.

Mrs. J. B. Edmonds (Jeanne)

For a moist and tender chicken, cook chicken pieces or whole chicken in cooking bags in oven with celery, onion, salt, and pepper for seasoning.

Chicken Florentine

1 (15-ounce) can artichoke hearts, quartered
1 (10-ounce) package frozen chopped spinach, thawed, drained, and squeezed dry
2 whole chicken breasts, cooked and cut into bite size pieces
1 (10¾-ounce) can cream of chicken soup

½ cup mayonnaise
1 tablespoon lemon juice
1 teaspoon curry powder
¾ cup shredded sharp cheddar cheese
1½ tablespoons butter, melted
½ cup dry breadcrumbs

- Preheat oven to 350 degrees.

- Line buttered 11x7x2-inch casserole dish with artichokes, then spinach. Sprinkle chicken over spinach.

- Combine soup, mayonnaise, lemon juice, and curry powder. Spread over casserole. Sprinkle with cheese. Top with buttered breadcrumbs.

- Bake 30 minutes or until hot, bubbly, and slightly brown Serves 8 to 10.

Mrs. J. Roy Bourgoyne (Helen Ruth)

Chicken Marengo

4 whole chicken breasts, skinned
4 tablespoons margarine
⅛ teaspoon garlic salt
1½ cups chicken bouillon
¼ cup white wine

3 large tomatoes, quartered
2 large onions, quartered
8 ounces fresh mushrooms, sliced
Cooked rice

- Brown chicken in margarine in deep skillet. Sprinkle with garlic salt and add remaining ingredients. Cover and simmer about 1 hour, adding more liquid if necessary.

- Before serving, remove meat from bones and return to skillet. Serve over rice. Serves 6.

Mrs. Michael J. Harty (Kay)

Chicken Indienne

Stuffing:
4 tablespoons butter
1 small onion, chopped
½ cup cooked rice

½ cup minced ham
½ tablespoon fines herbes
1 egg, beaten

- Melt butter, add onion and cook until soft.

- Add rice, ham, and fines herbes; blend with egg.

3½ pounds chicken
½ lemon
2 tablespoons butter
1 teaspoon curry powder

1 clove garlic, crushed
½ teaspoon salt
½ cup chicken broth

- Preheat oven to 350 degrees.

- Stuff chicken; sew the opening.

- Rub with cut lemon.

- Heat butter in baking dish — when foamy, add curry and garlic.

- Place chicken on its back, pour in stock and cover well.

- Bake 1 hour, turning 3 times while cooking.

Mrs. Lyle E. Muller (Mary)

Easy Chicken and Rice

3 cups cooked wild rice
1 (2 to 3 pound) whole chicken,
** cooked, boned and cubed**
1 (4-ounce) can mushrooms
1 (10¾-ounce) can cream of
** mushroom soup**

½ soup can milk
½ cup chopped pecans (optional)
1 (2¼-ounce) can black olives,
** drained and chopped (optional)**
½ cup shredded cheddar cheese

- Preheat oven to 350 degrees.

- Combine all ingredients except cheese. Place in 3-quart casserole dish. Bake 30 to 35 minutes, uncovered.

- Add cheese and return to oven for 10 minutes before serving. Serves 6 to 8.

Mrs. Mark E. Wiygul (Jan)

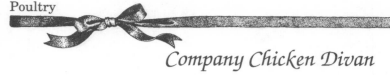

Company Chicken Divan

2 (10-ounce) packages frozen
  broccoli spears
1 (6-ounce) roll garlic cheese
2 tablespoons margarine
1 medium onion, chopped
1 (10¾-ounce) can mushroom soup
1 (8-ounce) carton sour cream

1 (4-ounce) can mushroom pieces
½ cup white wine
1 (2 pound) chicken, cooked, boned
  and chopped
½ cup breadcrumbs
½ cup chopped pecans

- Preheat oven to 350 degrees.

- Cook broccoli and drain. Place in 13x9x2-inch casserole dish. Slice garlic cheese in pieces over broccoli and set aside.

- In saucepan, heat margarine, add chopped onion and sauté. Add soup, sour cream, mushrooms, and wine. Cook until bubbly, stirring constantly. Add chicken pieces. Pour chicken mixture over broccoli and cheese. Sprinkle with breadcrumbs and pecans. Bake 30 to 40 minutes. Serve 6.

Mrs. Bruce H. McCullar (Jennifer)

Hot Chicken Salad I

1½ cups mayonnaise
1 (10¾-ounce) can cream of chicken
  soup
1 cup diced chicken, cooked
½ cup diced celery
½ (10-ounce) package frozen peas,
  cooked

2 or 3 hard-boiled eggs
Salt and pepper to taste
1 (3-ounce) can small chow mein
  noodles, well seasoned

- Preheat oven to 350 degrees.

- Combine mayonnaise and soup. Add chicken, celery, peas, and eggs. Salt and pepper to taste.

- Put noodles on top.

- Bake covered first 20 minutes, remove cover. Bake an additional 20 minutes. Serves 4 to 6.

Mrs. Lesley H. Binkley, Jr. (Nancy)

Hot Chicken Salad II

4 whole chicken breasts, cooked, drained and diced
¾ cup chopped celery
1½ cups shredded cheddar cheese
2 hard-boiled eggs, sliced
1 (10½-ounce) can cream of chicken soup
Salt and pepper to taste

1 (2¼-ounce) package slivered almonds
1 small onion, grated
¾ cup mayonnaise
½ cup chicken broth
1 small package potato chips, crushed

- Preheat oven to 350 degrees.

- Mix all ingredients together except potato chips.

- Put in greased 13x9x2-inch baking dish and top with crushed potato chips.

- Bake 30 minutes. Serves 4 to 6.

Mrs. Nathan R. Walley (Donna)

Karen's Chicken Soufflé

9 slices white bread, cut into pieces
4 cups cooked chicken, cubed
1 (8-ounce) can sliced mushrooms, drained
¼ cup margarine, melted
1 (8-ounce) can sliced water chestnuts, drained
8 ounces sharp cheddar cheese, shredded

½ cup mayonnaise
4 eggs, well beaten
2 cups milk
1 teaspoon salt
1 (10¾-ounce) can cream of mushroom soup
1 (2-ounce) jar chopped pimentos, drained
2 cups breadcrumbs

- Line a buttered 13x9x2-inch baking dish with bread. Cover with chicken.

- Sauté mushrooms in margarine and spoon over chicken. Add layers of water chestnuts and cheese.

- In separate bowl combine mayonnaise, eggs, milk, and salt. Beat well and pour over cheese.

- Combine soup and pimentos and pour over casserole. Cover with foil and refrigerate for 8 hours or overnight.

- Bake in 350 degree oven 30 minutes. Top with breadcrumbs and bake an additional 20 minutes.

Mrs. Bruce H. McCullar (Jennifer)

Louisiana Chicken Spaghetti for a Crowd

15 pounds fryers (breasts and
   thighs)
Water
1½ cups margarine
12 cups chopped celery
3 onions, chopped
3 green bell peppers, chopped
3 cloves garlic, minced
3 (10¾-ounce) cans tomato soup

3 (10¾-ounce) cans cream of
   mushroom soup
4 cups chicken broth
6 tablespoons chili powder
Salt and garlic salt to taste
2 pounds spaghetti
24 ounces pasteurized process
   cheese spread, cubed
Dash of cayenne (optional)

- Preheat oven to 350 degrees when ready to bake.

- Boil chicken in water to cover for 5 minutes; reduce heat and simmer until tender, approximately 2 hours.

- Remove chicken, bone, skin, and chop meat. Reserve broth.

- In large pan melt margarine and sauté chopped vegetables; add garlic. Stir in soups, broth and seasonings and simmer 45 minutes. Add chicken.

- Cook spaghetti; drain and mix with sauce and cheese. Season with cayenne. Bake in 3 (3-quart) casseroles 45 minutes. Serves 30.

Mrs. J. Thomas Cobb (Ann)

O'Farrell's Chicken Stew

1 chicken, cut up
5 cups water
2 to 3 ribs celery, chopped
½ medium onion, chopped
1 teaspoon salt
½ teaspoon pepper
2 cups cooked rice

2 medium potatoes, diced and
   cooked
4 chicken bouillon cubes
1 pound processed cheese
Paprika
Fresh parsley

- Boil chicken in water with celery, onion, salt and pepper 1 hour.

- Take chicken from water and remove skin and bone.

- Return meat to broth; add rice, potatoes, and bouillon cubes.

- Cut cheese into small pieces and add to soup. When cheese is melted, sprinkle with paprika and garnish with fresh parsley. Serves 6 to 8.

Dr. O'Farrell Shoemaker

Nanny's Chicken Pot Pie

4 chicken pieces (half breast, thigh, leg or wing)
Water
2 hard-boiled eggs, chopped
5 tablespoons cornstarch

2 cups chicken broth
Salt and pepper to taste
2 tablespoons butter or margarine
1 small tube (4 rolls) crescent rolls

- Boil chicken pieces in water until tender, reserving 2 cups broth. Remove chicken from bone.

- Preheat oven to 375 degrees.

- Place chicken in 1½-quart casserole. Sprinkle with chopped eggs.

- Mix cornstarch and broth; add salt, pepper, and butter; bring to boil and cook until thickened, stirring constantly. Pour thickened broth over chicken and eggs.

- Unroll dough and place on top of chicken mixture. Bake 12 minutes. Serves 2.

Canned biscuits may be used in place of crescent rolls.

Mrs. J. W. Breazeal (Sue)

Parmesan Chicken

2 cups round buttery cracker crumbs
¾ cup Parmesan cheese
¼ cup dry parsley flakes
¼ teaspoon garlic powder

¼ teaspoon pepper
10 chicken breast halves, skinned and boned
½ cup margarine, melted

- Preheat oven to 350 degrees.

- Mix crumbs, cheese, and seasonings.

- Dip chicken in margarine, then in crumbs. Place in 13x9x2-inch baking dish and dot with margarine.

- Bake 1 hour. Do not turn chicken. Serves 8 to 10.

Mrs. James G. Avery (Karen)

Southern Fried Chicken

3 cups vegetable oil
1½ cups flour
¼ teaspoon salt
¼ teaspoon pepper

¼ teaspoon paprika
1 chicken, fat and skin removed,
   cut into pieces
¾ cup buttermilk

- Heat oil in large iron skillet on medium heat until hot.

- Combine flour, salt, pepper, and paprika. Dip each chicken part in buttermilk then in flour mixture.

- Be sure oil is very hot before putting chicken pieces in, otherwise chicken will be greasy. Brown chicken approximately 10 minutes on each side with skillet covered. Remove cover and turn up heat to medium-high and cook chicken 5 minutes longer on each side. This is when the chicken becomes nice and crisp.

- Remove and drain well on paper towels. Serve hot or cold.

- Serves 6.

Mrs. Jack W. Hoelscher (Barbara)

Sweet and Sour Chicken

3 pound fryer or 8 split breasts
1 (8-ounce) bottle Russian, Casino,
   or Catalina dressing

2 envelopes dry onion soup mix
1 (8-ounce) jar apricot or peach jam

- Preheat oven to 300 degrees.

- Place chicken in 13x9x2-inch greased baking dish, skin side up.

- In separate bowl, mix remaining ingredients and spread over chicken. Bake covered 1 hour, then uncovered 1 hour. Serves 8.

Mrs. Joe L. Cannon (Nell)

Quick and Easy Chicken Delight

1 cup sour cream
1 (10¾-ounce) can mushroom soup
½ cup milk
2 (6½-ounce) cans Swanson's white
   chicken

1 cup chicken broth
½ cup margarine
1 (6-ounce) package cheddar cheese
   croutons

- Preheat oven to 350 degrees.

- Mix sour cream, mushroom soup, milk, and chicken. Pour into 2-quart casserole.

- Mix chicken broth and margarine. Heat until margarine melts. Add croutons and pour over chicken layer. Bake 45 minutes. Serves 4.

Variation: Breadcrumbs may be substituted for cheddar cheese croutons.

Dr. Robert K. Armstrong

Stuffed Cornish Hens with Apple Dressing

4 Cornish hens
3 cups cubed bread, toasted
¼ cup margarine, melted
½ cup chopped onions
½ cup chopped celery

4 tablespoons slivered almonds
½ teaspoon salt
¼ teaspoon black pepper
½ cup diced apple
¼ cup water

- Preheat oven to 400 degrees.

- Rinse and dry hens.

- Mix all ingredients in large bowl. Place ¼ dressing inside each hen. Sew the opening and pull drumsticks together.

- Cook hens 20 minutes at 400 degrees and then 50 minutes at 325 degrees. Serves 4 to 6.

Dr. Charles E. Harbison

Cornish Hens with Raspberry-Sesame Sauce

4 Cornish hens
2 tablespoons butter
¼ cup lime juice
¾ teaspoon salt

⅛ teaspoon white pepper
⅓ cup sesame seed, toasted
1 (10-ounce) jar raspberry jelly

- Preheat oven to 350 degrees.

- Remove giblets, rinse hens and pat dry.

- In saucepan, melt butter and add 2 tablespoons lime juice, salt and pepper. Brush hens inside and out with this mixture.

- Tie legs together and place on rack in roasting pan. Roast hens about 1 hour and 15 minutes, basting often with lime mixture.

- In small saucepan combine sesame seed, jelly, and remaining lime juice. Heat and stir until blended. Brush on hens the last 5 minutes of cooking.

- Serve the remaining raspberry-sesame sauce as a complement. Serves 4.

Mrs. James F. Bigger, Jr. (Pat)

Roast Turkey

Turkey
Poultry seasoning
1 onion

3 ribs celery
Butter or margarine

- Preheat oven to 450 degrees.

- Rub cleaned turkey inside and out with poultry seasoning. Place onion and celery in cavity. Rub outside with butter or margarine. Place on rack in roasting pan, breast side up, in oven. Reduce heat to 350 degrees immediately. Baste with pan drippings to which a small amount of water has been added to prevent burning and cook until tender — 20 minutes per pound if turkey weighs under 6 pounds and 15 minutes per pound if turkey weighs over 6 pounds.

- You may cover breast and leg tops with cheesecloth saturated in melted shortening to prevent drying.

Mrs. John Mallett Barron (Doy)

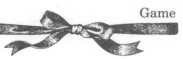

Dove Pie

1 small recipe of pastry
  (see index — Southern Pecan Pie)
Sage
20 to 35 dove breasts
1 to 2 cups red wine
1 tablespoon Worcestershire sauce
Salt, pepper, and seasoned salt to
  taste
½ teaspoon garlic salt
⅛ teaspoon red pepper
Water
3 large potatoes, peeled and diced

3 to 4 carrots, sliced
1 large onion, diced
1 (16-ounce) can tiny English peas
1 cup finely chopped green bell
  pepper
1 (10¾-ounce) can mushrooms
1 (10¾-ounce) can cream of mushroom or cream of chicken soup,
  undiluted
Kitchen Bouquet
Cornstarch, if needed

- Preheat oven to 300 degrees.

- Roll pastry and cut in desired shapes; sprinkle with sage. Bake and set aside.

- Place dove breasts in roaster. Add wine, Worcestershire, seasonings, and enough water to barely cover. Cook until tender.

- While still warm, remove meat from bones and place in 3-quart casserole. Add partially cooked vegetables and mushrooms.

- In saucepan, heat and stir 4 cups of broth from roaster. Add soup, seasoning to taste, Kitchen Bouquet, and cornstarch, if needed. Pour mixture over vegetables and doves.

- Cover with foil and bake 30 to 45 minutes until vegetables are tender but firm.

- Top with pastry cut outs and serve at once. Serves 10 to 12.

Mrs. James F. Bennett, Jr. (Ann)

If you prefer less game flavor, soak ducks overnight in refrigerator in salt water.

Dove Breasts Stroganoff

1 medium onion, chopped
2 tablespoons butter or margarine
12 to 18 doves
1 (10½-ounce) can cream of celery
  soup
1 (4-ounce) jar mushrooms

½ cup Sauterne
½ teaspoon oregano
½ teaspoon rosemary
Salt and pepper to taste
1 teaspoon brown bouquet sauce
1 cup sour cream

- Preheat oven to 325 degrees.

- Sauté onion in butter.

- Arrange doves in large skillet.

- Make sauce by combining all remaining ingredients, except sour cream.

- Bake doves in sauce 1¼ hours, turning occasionally. Stir in sour cream. Bake an additional 30 minutes. Serves 6 to 8.

Mrs. Justin D. Towner (Ginny)

Duck with Wild Rice

2 to 4 ducks
Salt and pepper to taste
1 (10-ounce) bottle Worcestershire
  sauce

Water
4 large onions, cubed
8 ribs celery
1 (6¼-ounce) box wild rice

- Preheat oven to 350 degrees.

- Place ducks in roaster. Season with salt and pepper. Pour entire bottle Worcestershire over ducks, adding enough water to cover. Place onions and celery on top of ducks.

- Cover and bake until meat falls away from bone.

- Bone and remove skin from ducks.

- Cook wild rice according to package directions.

- After rice is cooked, place rice and large pieces of duck on platter.

Drippings may be used for a thin gravy.

Dr. Kenneth M. Caldwell

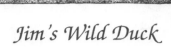

Jim's Wild Duck

3 wild ducks
Water
3 tablespoons soda
½ cup vinegar
2 tablespoons salt
1 potato, quartered
2 onions

Salt and pepper to taste
1 cooking apple, quartered
Celery leaves
1 orange, sliced
2 (11-ounce) cans mandarin oranges
Bacon slices
Wild rice, cooked

- Cover ducks with water, add soda, vinegar, and salt. Soak overnight in refrigerator.

- Before cooking, pour off water and add fresh water, potato, and 1 onion. Boil gently 45 minutes.

- Pour off water and wash duck thoroughly. Season cavity with salt and pepper. Insert quartered onion, apple, and celery leaves.

- Preheat oven to 275 degrees.

- Place duck in covered roaster in 1 inch water. Place slices of orange on each duck and pour mandarin oranges over breast. Top with bacon slice, salt and pepper.

- Bake 3½ hours, basting every 30 minutes. Remove cover last half hour. Serve with wild rice.

Good with Pear Chutney (see index).

Mrs. James F. Bennett, Jr. (Ann)

Quick and Easy Duck

1 (10¾-ounce) can cream of
  mushroom soup
3 tablespoons dried Lipton onion
  soup mix

½ cup sherry
2 whole ducks

- Preheat oven to 300 degrees.

- Combine soup, soup mix, and sherry.

- Place ducks in heavy aluminum foil and pour soup mixture over them. Seal tightly and bake 2½ to 3 hours. Serves 4.

Dr. Charles E. Harbison

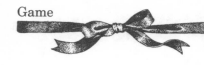

Smothered Quail

4 quail
Salt and pepper to taste
¼ cup butter
¾ cup white wine
⅛ teaspoon thyme

½ bay leaf
1 (10½-ounce) can condensed
  consommé
2 tablespoons flour

- Rub quail with salt and pepper, inside and out. Brown in butter.

- Add wine, thyme, bay leaf, and consommé; sprinkle flour over quail. Cover and simmer until tender, about 55 minutes.

- Spoon pan juices over quail when served. Yields 4 servings.

Mrs. John S. Cannon (Maggie)

Blender Béarnaise Sauce

2 tablespoons white wine
1 tablespoon tarragon vinegar
2 teaspoons chopped tarragon
2 teaspoons chopped shallots or
  onion
¼ teaspoon ground black pepper

½ cup butter
3 egg yolks
2 tablespoons lemon juice
¼ teaspoon salt
Pinch cayenne

- Combine wine, vinegar, tarragon, shallots, and pepper in saucepan. Boil rapidly until almost all liquid disappears.

- Heat butter to bubbling.

- Place egg yolks, lemon juice, salt, and cayenne in electric blender jar. Cover, turn on and off at high speed while adding butter in thin stream. Add herb mixture, blend on high again for a few seconds. Makes 1 cup.

Mrs. John Mallett Barron (Doy)

Spicy-Spicy Mustard

2 (2-ounce) cans Coleman's mustard
1 cup malt vinegar

3 eggs, beaten
½ cup sugar

- Combine mustard and vinegar. Leave overnight.

- Combine eggs and sugar. Add to mustard and vinegar mixture and cook in double boiler until thick.

- Refrigerate.

Mrs. James W. Clark (Carolyn)

Giblet Gravy

Turkey giblets (neck, liver, gizzard, heart)
1 medium onion, chopped
3 ribs celery, chopped
1 quart water

½ teaspoon salt
¼ teaspoon pepper
4 tablespoons butter
4 tablespoons flour
2 hard-boiled eggs, chopped

- Bring first 6 ingredients to boil in 2-quart saucepan. Reduce heat to low and cook until tender, about 1 to 2 hours.

- Remove meat from neck bones and chop liver, gizzard, and heart. Set aside.

- In saucepan, melt butter over medium heat, add flour, stirring constantly for 2 minutes. Add broth from giblets and cook until thickened. Add meat, chopped giblets, and eggs. Serve with turkey and cornbread dressing.

The first two steps may be followed the day before serving and refrigerated.

Mrs. John Mallett Barron (Doy)

Dry onion soup sprinkled over a roast which is to be sealed in foil will make a delicious gravy while the roast is cooking.

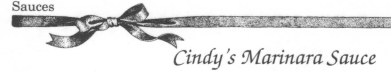

Cindy's Marinara Sauce

4 garlic cloves, minced
¼ cup olive oil
4 carrots, chopped
4 ribs celery, chopped
1 cup white wine
1 teaspoon basil

1 teaspoon oregano
1 teaspoon cayenne or to taste
2 (28-ounce) cans tomatoes
4 (15-ounce) cans tomato sauce
1 tablespoon brown sugar

• Sauté garlic in olive oil. Add carrots, celery, and wine; cook until wine is almost absorbed. Add spices, tomatoes, and tomato sauce.

• Bring to boil. Simmer at least 4 hours. Allow to cool.

Mrs. Cecil L. Raines (Ann)

Mint Sauce for Lamb

½ cup sugar
¼ cup white wine vinegar
¼ cup water

1 (10-ounce) jar mint jelly
1 cup finely chopped fresh mint
  leaves

• Mix sugar, vinegar, and water in saucepan and heat at medium temperature. When sugar dissolves, add jelly and simmer until jelly is completely melted. Add mint leaves and serve immediately. Serves 4 to 6.

Cookbook Committee

Wild Game Sauce

½ cup orange juice
½ cup grape juice
2 tablespoons currant jelly

Grated rind of 1 orange
1 teaspoon prepared mustard
Dash pepper

• Combine ingredients in saucepan and simmer for 5 to 6 minutes. (The consistency will not be thick.)

• Serve while warm over duck, quail, or turkey. Makes 1 cup.

Mrs. Frank J. Hudson (Bettye)

Orange Wine Sauce

⅔ cup sugar
3 tablespoons flour
2 eggs, beaten

3 cups orange juice
½ cup white wine

- Mix sugar and flour in double boiler. Add eggs, orange juice, and wine.
- Cook, stirring constantly, until thickened. Yields 4 cups.

Delicious served with sautéed shrimp or grilled chicken.

Mrs. Phillip Sherman, Jr. (Sandy)

Remoulade Sauce

6 egg yolks, cooked hard and grated
4 cloves garlic, finely chopped
3 tablespoons Creole mustard
4 tablespoons prepared mustard
4 cups mayonnaise
2 tablespoons paprika

3 tablespoons horseradish
2 tablespoons Worcestershire sauce
⅛ teaspoon Tabasco
4 tablespoons vinegar
4 tablespoons chopped parsley
Salt and pepper to taste

- Mix ingredients in large bowl.
- Refrigerate for 12 hours. Yields 1 quart.

Mrs. Dwight A. Morris (Cathy)

Sauce for Marshall Field Sandwich

1 clove garlic, minced
1 onion, grated
¼ cup chili sauce
¼ cup ketchup
1 cup mayonnaise
½ cup salad oil

1 teaspoon mustard
1 teaspoon Worcestershire sauce
Juice of 1 lemon
1 teaspoon pepper
1 teaspoon paprika

- Combine all ingredients. Serve over opened face sandwich layered in the following order: rye bread, ham, Swiss cheese, lettuce, sliced turkey, tomato, sliced boiled eggs, and bacon strips.

Cookbook Committee

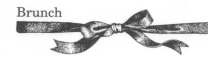

Eggs Whitney

2 English muffins, split and toasted
8 strips lean bacon, cooked and
  drained

4 eggs, poached
½ cup shredded cheddar cheese

- Preheat oven to 200 degrees.

- Place 2 strips bacon on each English muffin half. Top with well drained poached egg. Sprinkle with cheese.

- Warm in oven until cheese is slightly melted. Serves 2 to 4.

Dr. P. D. Miller, Jr.

Garlic Cheese Grits

1 cup quick cooking grits
1 (6-ounce) roll garlic cheese
½ cup butter

2 eggs, separated and beaten
¾ cup milk
Paprika

- Preheat oven to 375 degrees.

- Cook grits as package directs. Add cheese and butter. Cool.

- Combine egg yolks and milk. Pour grits in buttered 2-quart casserole and add milk and egg yolk mixture. Fold in beaten egg whites. Bake uncovered 1 hour. Dust top with paprika before serving. Serves 8.

Mrs. H. Franklin Miller (Carolyn)

Holiday Breakfast Casserole

1 pound sausage
4 to 5 slices French bread, cubed
2 cups grated sharp cheddar cheese
6 eggs

2½ cups milk
¾ teaspoon dry mustard
1 (10¾-ounce) can cream of
  mushroom soup

- Brown and drain sausage.

- Grease 13x9x2-inch baking dish.

- Scatter cubed bread over casserole bottom. Top with cheese and then sausage.

- Beat eggs with milk and dry mustard. Blend in soup. Pour over sausage.

- Cover and refrigerate at least 1 hour or overnight.

- Bake uncovered at 300 degrees 1 hour.

Mrs. Phillip Sherman, Sr. (Barbara)

Favorite Brunch Casserole

1 (16-ounce) package shredded
   sharp cheddar cheese
1 (4-ounce) can green chilies,
   chopped and drained

3 eggs, beaten
3 cups milk
1 cup biscuit baking mix
1 teaspoon salt

- Preheat oven to 350 degrees.

- Place half of shredded cheese into buttered 11x7x2-inch baking dish.

- Place chilies over cheese. Add remaining cheese.

- Beat eggs and add milk, baking mix, and salt. Stir to mix. Pour mixture over layers of chilies and cheese. Be sure cheese is completely covered.

- Bake 40 to 45 minutes.

- Serves 8.

Use mild or medium chilies, not hot!

Mrs. J. Roy Bourgoyne (Helen Ruth)

Deviled Eggs with Mushrooms

12 hard-boiled eggs
1 teaspoon salt
½ teaspoon curry powder
¼ teaspoon pepper
¼ teaspoon paprika

1 pound mushrooms, chopped
2 cups white sauce
½ cup buttered breadcrumbs
¼ cup shredded cheddar cheese

- Preheat oven to 400 degrees.

- Cut eggs in half lengthwise.

- Remove yolks and rub through a sieve. Add seasonings, some of the mushrooms, and just enough white sauce to hold mixture together. Refill egg whites with this mixture and press halves together.

- Place in 13x9x2-inch casserole and cover with white sauce mixed with remaining mushrooms.

- Sprinkle with buttered crumbs mixed with cheese. Bake approximately 20 minutes. Serve 6 generously.

Mrs. H. Franklin Miller (Carolyn)

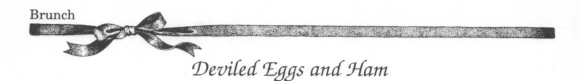

Deviled Eggs and Ham

6 hard-boiled eggs, cooled
2 tablespoons mayonnaise
½ teaspoon salt

½ teaspoon dry mustard
Dash white pepper

- Cut hard-boiled eggs in half, lengthwise. Carefully remove yolks.

- Mix yolks, mayonnaise, salt, mustard, and pepper. Stuff mixture into egg whites. Set aside.

White Sauce:
½ cup butter
¼ cup flour

2 cups milk

- In saucepan, melt butter and slowly stir in flour so mixture does not lump. Cook 1 minute on medium heat. Add milk and stir until mixture thickens.

1 cup shredded sharp cheddar cheese

1 cup English peas, drained
2 cups cooked ham, diced

- Add cheese, peas, and ham to white sauce; stir to mix.

- Preheat oven to 350 degrees.

- Line stuffed eggs into 13x9x2-inch casserole.

- Pour white sauce over eggs.

Topping:
½ cup buttered breadcrumbs

- Sprinkle top of casserole with breadcrumbs.

- Bake until hot and bubbly and crumbs are brown, about 20 minutes. Serves 8.

An unusual brunch dish and very good.

Mrs. C. Dale Moody Jr. (Doris)

Hash Brown Potato Casserole

1 (2-pound) package frozen hash
  brown potatoes, thawed
½ cup chopped onion
1 cup sour cream
1 (10¾-ounce) can cream of chicken
  soup

2 cups shredded cheddar cheese
1 teaspoon salt
1 teaspoon pepper
¼ cup melted butter or margarine
2 cups corn flake crumbs, crushed

• Preheat oven to 375 degrees.

• In large bowl, mix potatoes, onion, sour cream, soup, cheese, salt, and pepper.

• Place in greased 13x9x2-inch baking dish.

• In small bowl, toss melted butter and corn flake crumbs. Top casserole with buttered crumbs.

• Bake uncovered 45 minutes.

• Serves 12.

Cracker crumbs may be substituted for corn flake crumbs.

Mrs. Thomas H. Shipmon (Betty)
Mrs. Chester Lloyd (Betty)

Cheese Soufflé

5 slices white bread, buttered
1 teaspoon salt
1 teaspoon dry mustard
8 ounces sharp cheddar cheese,
  shredded

4 eggs
2 cups milk

• Cut each slice buttered bread into 16 cubes.

• Mix salt and dry mustard together.

• Butter 1½-quart casserole dish. Line casserole dish with bread cubes. Sprinkle with salt and mustard mixture. Cover with shredded cheese.

• In small mixing bowl, beat eggs. Add milk and stir. Pour mixture over cheese and bread.

• Refrigerate 4 or 5 hours or overnight.

• Bake 1 hour in 350 degree oven. Serves 6 to 8.

Mrs. Kimbrough Boren (Pat)

Sausage Cheese Crescent Squares

1 can crescent rolls
8 ounces mild or hot sausage
1 (8-ounce) package shredded
  Monterey Jack cheese
4 eggs, slightly beaten
¾ cup milk

½ teaspoon salt
½ teaspoon pepper
¼ teaspoon oregano
2 tablespoons finely chopped green
  bell pepper

- Preheat oven to 425 degrees.

- Unroll crescent rolls and press into 13x9x2-inch baking pan.

- Cook and drain sausage. Sprinkle sausage and cheese on top of rolls.

- Mix beaten eggs, milk, salt, pepper, oregano, and chopped pepper. Pour over rolls and sausage layer. Bake 20 to 25 minutes.

- To serve for brunch, cut into 8 squares. To serve as appetizer, cut into 1-inch squares.

Mrs. William R. Priester, III (Jean)

Sausage Grits Casserole

1 cup 3-minute grits
3 cups canned undiluted beef
  bouillon
½ teaspoon salt
1 pound hot sausage

1 cup butter or margarine
4 eggs, beaten
1 cup milk
½ cup shredded cheddar cheese,
  divided

- Preheat oven to 350 degrees.

- Cook grits in bouillon and salt until thick (about 3 or 4 minutes).

- In skillet, cook sausage until well done. Drain on paper towels. Add sausage to cooked grits, mixing thoroughly.

- Add to mixture 1 cup margarine, beaten eggs, milk, and ¼ cup cheese.

- Pour into 2-quart casserole and sprinkle ¼ cup cheese on top.

- Bake 40 to 45 minutes, uncovered.

- Serves 8.

This looks very soupy before cooking; thickens as it bakes.

Mrs. John Mallett Barron (Doy)

Sausage Rice Casserole

2 pounds sausage
½ green bell pepper, seeded and
  chopped
1 large onion, chopped
1 cup chopped celery
6 cups water

2 packages (1 box) Lipton's chicken
  noodle soup mix
1 (5-ounce) can water chestnuts,
  sliced and drained
1 cup uncooked rice
½ cup slivered almonds

- Preheat oven to 350 degrees.

- Grease two 11x7x2-inch baking dishes.

- In large skillet, cook sausage about 3 minutes.

- Add bell pepper, onion, and celery. Cook until vegetables are soft and sausage is brown and crumbly. Drain well and set aside.

- In large bowl, mix water, soup mix, water chestnuts, and uncooked rice. Add sausage mixture. Stir and mix.

- Pour into two casserole dishes. Cover tightly and bake 30 minutes.

- Remove covers and sprinkle almonds on top. Bake uncovered 30 more minutes.

At the end of first 30 minutes, I cool one casserole and freeze for later use. Be sure to tape cooking directions on dish to be frozen.

Mrs. J. Roy Bourgoyne (Helen Ruth)

Sausage Surprise

1 (5-ounce) package medium size
  egg noodles
1 pound hot sausage
2 medium onions, chopped
1 (10¾-ounce) can mushroom soup

1 (10¾-ounce) can cheddar cheese
  soup
1 (13-ounce) can evaporated milk
1 (4-ounce) can mushroom pieces,
  drained

- Preheat oven to 350 degrees.

- Cook noodles according to package directions. Drain

- Cook sausage and onions until sausage is brown and crumbly. Drain well.

- Mix soups and milk together until smooth. Add mushrooms and stir.

- Add sausage and noodles; mix thoroughly.

- Place in greased 11x7x2-inch baking dish. Bake uncovered 35 to 40 minutes. Serves 6 to 8.

Mrs. Richard C. Harris (Beverly)

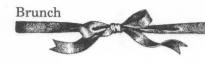

Bacon Quiche

12 slices bacon
1 cup shredded Swiss or Monterey
　Jack cheese
⅓ cup chopped onion
2 cups milk

½ cup biscuit baking mix
4 eggs
¼ teaspoon salt
½ teaspoon pepper

- Preheat oven to 350 degrees.

- Cook bacon crisp and drain well. Crumble.

- Grease 9 or 10-inch pie pan. Sprinkle crumbled bacon, cheese, and onion in bottom of pie pan.

- Place milk, biscuit mix, eggs, salt, and pepper in blender. Cover and blend on high 1 minute. Pour over ingredients in pie pan.

- Bake 50 to 55 minutes or until knife inserted in center comes out clean.

- Let stand a few minutes before serving. Serves 6 to 8.

Mrs. Jack E. Wells (Genie)

Dieters' Spinach Quiche

1 (10-ounce) package frozen
　chopped spinach
4 slices bacon, cooked crisp and
　crumbled
1 (9-inch) unbaked pie shell
4 eggs, beaten
4 cups skim milk

¼ cup finely chopped onion
½ teaspoon salt
¼ teaspoon paprika
½ teaspoon dry mustard
1¼ cups shredded cheddar cheese
　(reserve ¼ cup)

- Preheat oven to 400 degrees.

- Cook spinach according to package directions and drain well.

- Place drained spinach and crumbled bacon into pie shell.

- In large bowl, with electric mixer on medium, beat eggs and milk together. To the milk and eggs, add chopped onion, salt, paprika, dry mustard, and 1 cup cheese. Stir to mix. Pour over spinach and bacon in pie shell. Sprinkle with remaining ¼ cup cheese.

- Bake 40 minutes, or until set. Serves 6.

- Let set a few minutes before serving.

Mrs. James H. Thomas (Martha)

Vegetables
and
Side Dishes

Asparagus Soufflé

4 eggs
1 (15½-ounce) can asparagus
  spears, drained
1 cup shredded cheddar cheese

1 cup mayonnaise
1 (10¾-ounce) cream of mushroom
  soup
Dash Tabasco

- Preheat oven to 350 degrees.

- Beat eggs in blender. Add remaining ingredients and blend.

- Pour into lightly greased 1½-quart soufflé dish. Place soufflé dish in second pan and add 2-inches water. Bake 55 to 60 minutes or until knife inserted in center comes out clean. Serves 6.

Soufflé may be baked and served in small individual ramekins if preferred. Adjust baking time accordingly.

Mrs. Ernest H. Sigman, Jr. (Doris)

Asparagus Casserole

2 (10½-ounce) cans asparagus tips,
  drained with ¾ cup liquid
  reserved
1 cup cream of mushroom soup
2 tablespoons butter or margarine
6 ounces cheddar cheese, shredded

1 tablespoon Worcestershire sauce
4 tablespoons butter or margarine,
  melted
1½ cups cracker crumbs
½ cup chopped toasted almonds

- Preheat oven to 350 degrees.

- Combine asparagus liquid, soup, butter, cheese and Worcestershire in saucepan. Heat until well blended. Set aside.

- Combine melted butter, cracker crumbs and almonds.

- Alternate asparagus tips, sauce and crumbs in buttered 11x7x2-inch baking dish. Repeat layers. Bake 30 minutes. Serves 6 to 8.

Mrs. J. Garland Cherry, Jr. (Carol)

Elegant Green Bean Casserole

½ cup butter or margarine
2 (4-ounce) cans mushrooms, drained
1 medium onion, chopped
¼ cup flour
2 cups milk
1 cup half-and-half
2 cups shredded sharp cheddar cheese
⅛ teaspoon Tabasco
½ teaspoon salt
½ teaspoon pepper
4 (16-ounce) cans whole green beans, drained
1 (8-ounce) can water chestnuts, drained and sliced
1 (4-ounce) package sliced almonds

- Preheat oven to 375 degrees.

- Heat butter or margarine and sauté mushrooms and onion; add flour and cook until smooth. Add milk, half-and-half, cheese and seasonings; stir constantly and do not boil.

- Mix in beans and water chestnuts. Pour into two 11x7x2-inch baking dishes. Sprinkle almonds on top. Bake 30 minutes. Serves 10 to 12.

Freezes beautifully.

Mrs. Frank J. Hudson (Bettye)

Bean Bundles

1 (16-ounce) can whole green beans, drained
6 to 7 pieces bacon
French or Russian dressing

- Preheat oven to 350 degrees.

- Wrap 5 or 6 beans with ⅓ slice of bacon, making a bundle. Place in 11x7x2-inch baking dish with seam side down. Cover with French or Russian dressing.

- Bake uncovered 45 minutes or until bacon is done. Makes 18 to 20 bundles. Serves 6 to 8.

Mrs. J. Roy Bourgoyne (Helen Ruth)

Gladys Brinckerhoff's Beans

2 (10-ounce) packages frozen baby
  lima beans
Salted water
1 (14-ounce) can bean sprouts,
  drained
2 (6½-ounce) cans sliced water
  chestnuts, drained

2 (10¾-ounce) cans mushroom soup
⅛ teaspoon seasoned salt
¾ to 1 cup crushed Ritz crackers
2 tablespoons margarine, melted

- Preheat oven to 325 degrees.

- Cook lima beans in salted water until slightly done. Drain. Add bean sprouts, water chestnuts, soup, and salt. Place in greased 11x7x2-inch baking dish and top with cracker crumbs tossed in margarine. Bake 35 to 45 minutes. Serves 8.

Mrs. Bettie Campbell

Baked Beans Supreme

1 (28-ounce) can pork and beans
1 (15¼-ounce) can crushed pineapple, drained, and liquid reserved
1¼ cups diced ham

⅔ cup dark brown sugar
½ cup ketchup
2 teaspoons prepared mustard
½ teaspoon salt
4 to 6 slices bacon

- Preheat oven to 350 degrees.

- Combine beans, drained pineapple, and ham in large mixing bowl.

- In separate bowl, combine brown sugar, half of the pineapple juice, ketchup, prepared mustard, and salt. Mix with beans. Pour into 2-quart casserole. Top with bacon.

- Bake uncovered 1½ hours. Reduce heat to 300 degrees for another 45 minutes. Serves 6 to 8.

Mrs. Harold P. Thomas (Evelyn)

Barbecued Baked Beans

1 pound bacon, cut in thirds
1 large onion, finely chopped
5 (16-ounce) cans pork and beans
1 (14-ounce) bottle ketchup
2¼ cups brown sugar, packed

¼ cup mustard
¼ cup Worcestershire sauce
2 teaspoons liquid smoke
⅛ teaspoon red pepper (optional)

- Fry bacon in a 4 to 6-quart pot until crisp. Drain all but a small amount of the drippings.

- Add onion and sauté until clear. Add beans; stir well.

- Add ketchup, brown sugar, mustard, Worcestershire, liquid smoke, and pepper. Stir well. Lower heat to simmer. Cook until desired consistency, about 2 hours. Serves 20.

Mrs. Stephen Weir (Dottie)

Spicy Beets

1 (15-ounce) can beets, grated or shredded
1 tablespoon cornstarch
3 tablespoons sugar

½ teaspoon salt
2 tablespoons vinegar
1 tablespoon butter
2 tablespoons prepared horseradish

- Preheat oven to 350 degrees.

- Drain beets, reserving juice.

- Combine beet juice, cornstarch, sugar, salt, and vinegar; boil one minute. Add butter, horseradish, and beets. Bake in 1-quart covered casserole 30 minutes. Serves 4 to 6.

Mrs. J. Roy Bourgoyne (Helen Ruth)

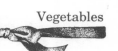

Scalloped Broccoli Casserole

2 (10-ounce) packages frozen
chopped broccoli, thawed
1 (4-ounce) can sliced mushrooms,
undrained
1 medium onion, chopped
½ cup margarine
1 (10¾-ounce) can cream of
mushroom soup

1 (6-ounce) roll garlic cheese
1 (2-ounce) package slivered
almonds
½ cup breadcrumbs
2 tablespoons margarine, melted

- Preheat oven to 350 degrees.

- Combine uncooked broccoli and mushrooms.

- Sauté onion in margarine and add to broccoli and mushrooms. Cook until partially done.

- Add soup and cheese, broken in pieces. Stir in almonds. Pour into buttered 3-quart casserole.

- Sprinkle breadcrumbs tossed in melted margarine on top. Bake 30 to 40 minutes or until bubbly. Serves 8 to 10.

Variation: Substitute ½ pound Velveeta cheese for garlic cheese roll.

Mrs. Billy W. McCann (Betty)
Mrs. Hilbert Nease (Betty)

Aunt Dot's Lemon Carrots

½ cup butter
½ cup sugar
2 teaspoons grated lemon peel

1 tablespoon lemon juice
24 small carrots, cooked

- Melt butter and sugar. Stir in lemon peel and juice.

- Add cooked carrots and simmer, stirring often until well glazed. Serves 6.

Mrs. Stephen Weir (Dottie)

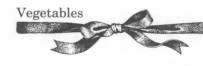

Carrot Pudding

**1 pound carrots, cooked and
  mashed**
½ cup sugar
1 cup milk
¼ teaspoon cinnamon

3 eggs, slightly beaten
¼ cup margarine, melted
3 tablespoons flour
1 teaspoon baking powder

- Preheat oven to 350 degrees.

- Mix ingredients. Pour into buttered 1½-quart casserole. Bake 1 hour. Serves 4
  to 6.

Mrs. James N. McLaughlin (Gwenice)

Baked Orange Glazed Carrots

**2 pounds carrots, cut into 3-inch
  pieces**
¼ cup firmly packed brown sugar
½ teaspoon ground cinnamon

1 tablespoon grated orange rind
½ cup orange juice
1 tablespoon butter, melted
1 cup water

- Preheat oven to 350 degrees.

- Place carrots on large sheet of foil and sprinkle brown sugar, cinnamon, and
  grated orange rind over carrots. Fold sides of foil up and add orange juice and
  butter. Fold and seal foil.

- Place in shallow pan with 1 cup water. Bake 45 to 60 minutes until tender.
  Serves 8.

Mrs. William F. Slagle (Shannon)

Corn Soufflé

2 tablespoons butter, melted
2 tablespoons flour
½ cup half-and-half or 2% milk
2½ cups cream style corn
1 teaspoon sugar

2 eggs, separated (or 2 egg beaters
   plus 1 egg white)
Salt and pepper to taste
2 tablespoons chopped pimento
   (optional)

• Preheat oven to 350 degrees.

• Melt butter in saucepan; add flour, stir slowly until blended. Add cream and stir until smooth and hot.

• Stir in corn and add sugar. Reduce heat to simmer.

• Remove small amount of corn mixture from pan and stir into well beaten egg yolks. Stir this into entire corn mixture and simmer several minutes. Add seasonings and remove from heat.

• Beat egg whites until stiff and fold lightly into corn mixture. Add pimento if desired. Pour into 2-quart greased casserole dish. Bake 30 minutes. Serves 4.

Freezes well before baking.

Mrs. William F. Slagle (Shannon)

Corn Custard

2 packages frozen cream style corn,
   thawed
3 tablespoons flour
3 tablespoons sugar
½ teaspoon mace

1 teaspoon salt
6 eggs, beaten
2 cups half-and-half or milk
¼ cup margarine, melted

• Preheat oven to 350 degrees.

• Mix all ingredients. Pour into greased 2-quart baking dish.

• Bake 1 hour or until knife inserted in center comes out clean. Serves 8.

This custard is just as good reheated the following day.

Mrs. L. C. Templeton (Virginia)

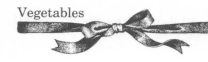

Corn Casserole

1 large onion, chopped
1 medium green bell pepper,
   chopped
2 tablespoons oil
1 (14-ounce) can cream style corn
1 (14-ounce) can whole kernel corn,
   drained
1 egg, beaten

1 (2-ounce) jar pimentos
⅔ cup milk
1 cup cracker crumbs
1 cup shredded cheddar cheese
¼ cup margarine, melted
2 tablespoons sugar
Salt, pepper, and red pepper to
   taste

- Preheat oven to 350 degrees.

- Sauté onion and bell pepper in oil. Add remaining ingredients.

- Place in greased 11x7x2-inch baking dish. Bake 30 minutes. Serves 10.

Mrs. J. B. Edmonds (Jeanne)

Eggplant Parmesan

1 large eggplant, peeled and sliced
   in ¼-inch slices
Salt
3 eggs
¼ cup milk

½ to 1 cup flour
Cooking oil
2 cups shredded mozzarella cheese
1 (15-ounce) jar spaghetti sauce
Grated Parmesan cheese

- Preheat oven to 350 degrees.

- Sprinkle eggplant with salt and let stand 15 minutes.

- Beat eggs and milk together; coat slices in flour, egg mixture, then flour again.

- Fry eggplant and drain. Layer eggplant, mozzarella cheese, and spaghetti sauce in
  11x7x2-inch baking dish. Top with Parmesan cheese. Bake 45 minutes or until
  bubbly. Serves 6.

Mrs. Robert L. Gardino (Ann)
Mrs. Huel M. Culbreath (Sue)

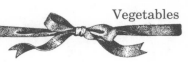

Eggplant Supreme

1 medium eggplant
Salted water
½ cup milk
1 onion, chopped

½ cup herb dressing, buttered
1 egg, beaten
2 tablespoons butter, melted
1 (8-ounce) jar Cheese Whiz

- Preheat oven to 350 degrees.

- Pare eggplant, cut into 1-inch cubes, and boil in salted water 8 minutes. Drain well.

- Add remaining ingredients. Place in greased 1-quart casserole. Bake 30 to 40 minutes. Serves 6.

Mrs. Ralph Braden (Virginia)

Buffet Mixed Vegetables

Sauce:
4 hard-boiled eggs, finely chopped
1 small onion, chopped
1 teaspoon salt
1 teaspoon paprika

1 cup mayonnaise
1 teaspoon Worcestershire
1 teaspoon prepared mustard
¼ teaspoon Tabasco

- Mix ingredients for sauce and set aside.

Vegetables:
1 (14-ounce) can English peas
1 (14-ounce) can lima beans

1 (14-ounce) can French style
  or cut green beans

- Heat vegetables and drain. Mix vegetables with sauce. Serve immediately. Serves 8 to 10.

Mrs. Billy W. McCann (Betty)

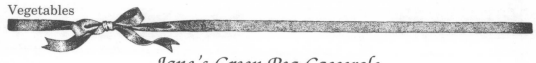

Jane's Green Pea Casserole

1 cup chopped onion
1 cup chopped green bell pepper
1 cup chopped celery
½ cup margarine
2 (15-ounce) cans tiny English peas, drained
1 (10¾-ounce) can mushroom soup

1 (8-ounce) can water chestnuts, drained and chopped
1 (3½-ounce) jar pimentos, drained and chopped
Salt and pepper to taste
Buttered breadcrumbs

- Preheat oven to 350 degrees.

- Sauté onion, bell pepper, and celery in margarine until soft.

- Combine all ingredients in 11x7x2-inch baking dish. Top with buttered bread crumbs. Bake uncovered 30 minutes. Serves 8 to 10.

Miss Traci Sherman

Mashed Potato Casserole

8 Irish or red potatoes, peeled, cooked and mashed
1 (8-ounce) package cream cheese

½ cup butter
1 cup sour cream
Salt and pepper to taste

- Preheat oven to 350 degrees.

- Combine all ingredients. Bake in 2-quart casserole uncovered 30 minutes. Serves 8.

Freezes well.

Mrs. Phillip Sherman, Jr. (Sandy)

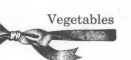

My Sister's Potatoes

1 (32-ounce) package frozen hash browns, thawed
4 tablespoons butter or margarine, melted
½ cup chopped onion
1 cup sour cream
1 (10¾-ounce) can cream of chicken soup
2 cups shredded cheddar cheese
1 teaspoon salt
1 teaspoon pepper
2 cups cornflake crumbs, tossed with butter or margarine

- Preheat oven to 375 degrees.

- Mix all ingredients except cornflake crumbs.

- Pour into greased 13x9x2-inch baking dish. Top with buttered crumbs. Bake 45 minutes. Serves 12.

Mrs. N. Edward Tillman (Ann)
Mrs. Bruce H. McCullar (Jennifer)

Cheesy Stuffed Potatoes

4 medium baking potatoes
½ cup butter or margarine
½ cup half-and-half
1 teaspoon salt
⅛ teaspoon cayenne
½ medium onion, finely chopped
1 cup shredded sharp cheddar cheese
½ teaspoon paprika

- Preheat oven to 375 degrees.

- Bake potatoes until fork pierces easily. Cut potatoes in half lengthwise. Scoop out potatoes and whip with butter, cream, salt, cayenne, onion, and cheese.

- Refill shells. Sprinkle with paprika and reheat at 450 degrees 15 minutes. Serves 8.

These freeze well.

Variation: Add 1 (6½-ounce) can crabmeat.

Mrs. O'Farrell Shoemaker (Melanie)
Mrs. Jack E. Wells (Genie)

Super Duper Potatoes

9 large red potatoes
½ cup butter
2 cups half-and-half

1 tablespoon salt
8 ounces sharp cheddar cheese,
  shredded

- Boil potatoes, drain, and chill. Peel and grate potatoes.

- Preheat oven to 350 degrees.

- Melt butter, and half-and-half and salt. Mix with potatoes and cheese. Pour into 2-quart casserole. Bake 1 hour. Serves 8.

Freezes well.

Miss Traci Sherman
Mrs. Justin D. Towner (Ginny)

Tortellini

1 (12-ounce) package Louisa brand
  tortellini
¼ cup margarine or butter
3 to 4 green onions, chopped
8 ounces mushrooms, sliced

1 (16-ounce) can artichoke hearts,
  quartered and drained
2 zucchini, sliced
½ cup grated Parmesan cheese
½ cup whipping cream

- Prepare tortellini according to directions.

- Melt margarine and sauté onions, mushrooms, artichoke hearts, and zucchini. Mix with tortellini. Add cheese and cream and toss. Serve immediately in 13x9x2-inch baking dish. If prepared ahead, heat 20 to 30 minutes in 350 degree oven. Serves 10 to 12.

Mrs. Justin D. Towner (Ginny)

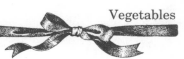

Holiday Sweet Potatoes

6 cups cooked and mashed sweet potatoes
1½ cups sugar

1½ teaspoons vanilla
¾ cup butter, melted

• Preheat oven to 350 degrees.

• Mix all ingredients and pour into greased 2-quart baking dish.

Topping:
1½ cups brown sugar
1½ cups chopped pecans

⅓ cup flour
⅓ cup soft butter

• Combine all ingredients and sprinkle on top of sweet potato mixture. Bake 45 minutes. Serves 6 to 8.

Mrs. W. L. Burgess, Jr. (Delores)
Mrs. James G. Avery (Karen)

Sweet Potato Casserole

5 to 6 sweet potatoes
¼ cup butter
¼ teaspoon cinnamon
⅛ teaspoon nutmeg

½ cup orange juice
3 tablespoons brown sugar
½ teaspoon vanilla
½ cup miniature marshmallows

• Preheat oven to 350 degrees.

• Bake sweet potatoes until soft, 45 minutes to 1 hour. Let potatoes cool slightly, peel and mash.

• Add butter, cinnamon, nutmeg, orange juice, brown sugar, and vanilla. Pour into greased 1½-quart casserole.

• Top with marshmallows and bake approximately 30 minutes. Serves 6 to 8.

Mrs. Phillip Sherman, Jr. (Sandy)

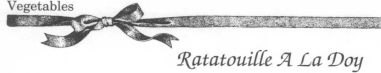

Ratatouille A La Doy

1 medium eggplant, peeled and sliced	2 tablespoons basil
3 small zucchini, sliced	1 tablespoon Italian herb seasoning
1 large onion, sliced	Freshly ground black pepper, to taste
Olive oil	Garlic to taste or garlic powder
1 (14½-ounce) can stewed tomatoes	

- Sauté vegetables in olive oil in heavy Dutch oven. Add remaining ingredients, cover, and simmer 1 hour, stirring occasionally. Remove lid and continue cooking to reduce liquid if necessary. Serves 6 to 8.

Mrs. John Mallett Barron (Doy)

Rice Stodge

4 cups cooked rice	2 slightly beaten eggs
1 cup parsley, minced	1 teaspoon salt
4 ounces cheddar cheese, shredded	⅛ teaspoon pepper
1 medium onion, chopped	3 tablespoons butter, melted
2 cups milk	

- Preheat oven to 375 degrees.

- Combine all ingredients, except butter.

- Put in buttered 2½-quart casserole. Drizzle melted butter on top. Bake 40 minutes. Serves 10.

Mrs. Vernon Reed (Billye)

Rice with Pine Nuts

1 cup butter	½ cup pine nuts
1 cup Uncle Ben's long grain rice	3 cups hot chicken or beef broth

- Melt butter in heavy skillet. Add rice and pine nuts. Sauté until golden brown.

- Pour in hot broth and cook for 2 minutes only.

- Remove from heat and cover 1 hour. Serves 6.

Mrs. James G. Sousoulas (Sophie)

Company Rice Casserole

½ cup butter or margarine, melted
1 cup uncooked rice
1 (10¾-ounce) can chicken broth
1 (10¾-ounce) can onion soup
1 (4-ounce) can mushrooms,
  drained

1 (2-ounce) jar chopped pimentos
1 cup shredded cheddar cheese
1 (2-ounce) package slivered
  almonds
Garlic salt and pepper to taste

- Preheat oven to 350 degrees.

- Melt butter or margarine in 1½-quart casserole. Add remaining ingredients.

- Cover and cook 1½ hours. Serves 6 to 8.

Variation: 1 (8-ounce) can sliced water chestnuts, drained, instead of almonds.

Mrs. L. Carl Anderson (Maxine)
Mrs. James B. Cochran (Linda)

Spanish Rice

½ cup vegetable oil
1 cup chopped onion
¾ cup chopped green bell pepper
½ cup uncooked rice

2 teaspoons salt
½ teaspoon pepper
1 (28-ounce) can tomatoes
1 small bay leaf

- Preheat oven to 350 degrees.

- Mix ingredients and pour into 2-quart casserole. Cover and bake 1 hour and 15 minutes, stirring occasionally. Serves 4 to 6.

This is very good served with all Mexican food.

Mrs. George H. Bouldien (Judy)

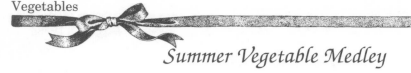

Summer Vegetable Medley

2 pounds new potatoes, scrubbed
  well
Water
1¼ teaspoons salt
½ teaspoon ground basil
1 cup cherry tomatoes
1 pound zucchini, sliced

½ pound summer squash, sliced
⅛ teaspoon freshly ground black
  pepper
2 tablespoons butter
¼ cup half-and-half
Fresh parsley, for garnish

- Place potatoes in saucepan with ½-inch boiling water and salt; cover, and boil 15 minutes. Shake pan occasionally. Add basil and tomatoes; cook 5 more minutes.

- In separate pan, cook sliced zucchini and squash about 12 minutes. Combine with potatoes. Add pepper, butter, and cream. Heat a few seconds.

- Turn into a serving dish and garnish with parsley. Serve immediately. Serves 6.

Mrs. William F. Slagle (Shannon)

Mexican Squash

5 to 8 medium yellow squash
4 tablespoons chopped onion
6 tablespoons butter or margarine,
  divided
1½ cups shredded cheddar cheese

1 (10-ounce) can Rotel tomatoes and
  green chilies
Salt and pepper to taste
¾ cup coarsely ground cracker
  crumbs

- Preheat oven to 350 degrees.

- Peel and slice squash; cook with chopped onion until tender.

- Drain squash and add 4 tablespoons butter, cheese, tomatoes and green chilies, salt, and pepper. Stir lightly. Place in buttered 2-quart casserole.

- Top with crumbs tossed in remaining 2 tablespoons melted butter. Bake 30 minutes or until bubbly. Serves 6 to 8.

*Freezes beautifully. Better if made a day ahead
to give flavors a chance to blend.*

Mrs. J. Garland Cherry, Jr. (Carol)

Thanksgiving Squash

3 cups yellow squash, sliced
Salted water
½ cup chopped onion
6 tablespoons butter or margarine, divided
1 (10¾-ounce) can cream of chicken soup

1 carrot, grated
1 cup sour cream
⅛ teaspoon pepper
1 (8-ounce) package herb dressing

- Preheat oven to 350 degrees.

- Cook squash in salted water, drain well, and mash.

- Sauté onion in 2 tablespoons butter. Mix squash, onion, soup, carrot, sour cream, and pepper.

- Melt 4 tablespoons butter and add to dressing. Put half the dressing in bottom of 11x7x2-inch baking dish. Add squash mixture.

- Top with remaining dressing. Bake 30 minutes or until bubbly. Serves 10 to 12.

Mrs. Joe L. Cannon (Nell)

Squash and Apple Bake

2 acorn or butternut squash
1 (20-ounce) can pie sliced apples
2 tablespoons cornstarch
¾ cup dark corn syrup
2 tablespoons margarine

1 teaspoon lemon juice
¾ teaspoon nutmeg
½ teaspoon salt
¼ cup chopped pecans

- Preheat oven to 350 degrees.

- Cut squash in half and remove seeds. Bake cut side down in shallow pan for 30 to 40 minutes. Cool slightly and peel. Cut into slices.

- Drain apples, reserving liquid. Mix apples and squash and place in 13x9x2-inch baking dish.

- Blend reserved juice and cornstarch in saucepan and stir in next five ingredients. Cook and stir until thick and bubbly. Pour over squash and apples. Sprinkle with nuts. Bake 25 to 30 minutes. Serves 6 to 8.

Mrs. Vernon Reed (Billye)

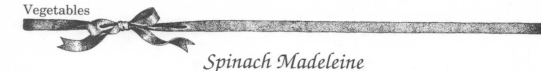

Spinach Madeleine

2 (10-ounce) packages frozen
  chopped spinach
4 tablespoons butter or margarine
2 tablespoons flour
2 tablespoons chopped onion
½ cup evaporated milk
1 cup vegetable liquid
½ teaspoon salt

½ teaspoon pepper
½ teaspoon celery salt
½ teaspoon garlic powder
1 teaspoon Worcestershire sauce
Red pepper to taste
1 (6-ounce) roll jalapeño cheese,
  cubed
Breadcrumbs (optional)

- Cook spinach; drain well, saving liquid.

- Melt butter over low heat. Add flour, stirring until blended. Add onion and cook until soft.

- Blend in milk and spinach liquid slowly, stirring constantly, until smooth and thick. Add seasonings and cheese, stirring until cheese melts. Combine with spinach.

- This may be served immediately as a dip or put into a 2-quart casserole, topped with breadcrumbs, and refrigerated overnight.

- Bake 30 minutes in 350 degree oven. Serves 6.

Mrs. Winfield Dunn (Betty)

Spinach New Orleans

3 (10-ounce) packages spinach,
  cooked and drained
1 (8-ounce) package cream cheese
2 tablespoons butter or margarine
Grated rind of 1 lemon
1 tablespoon lemon juice

Salt and pepper to taste
1 cup Pepperidge Farm herb
  dressing mix
2 tablespoons butter or margarine,
  melted

- Preheat oven to 350 degrees.

- Combine the first 6 ingredients and pour into well greased 11x7x2-inch casserole.

- Top with dressing mix and butter combined. Bake 20 minutes. Serves 8.

Mrs. James W. Clark (Carolyn)

Spinach Supreme

3 (10-ounce) packages frozen
  chopped spinach
1 (10¾-ounce) can cream of celery
  soup
½ green bell pepper, chopped
1 egg, beaten
2 slices bread, torn into small
  pieces

¼ cup milk
2 teaspoons minced onion
Salt and pepper to taste
1 teaspoon garlic salt
1 (13¾-ounce) can artichoke hearts,
  drained and mashed
½ cup grated Parmesan cheese
3 tablespoons butter or margarine

- Preheat oven to 350 degrees.

- Cook and drain spinach. Add soup, bell pepper, egg, bread, milk, onion, salt, pepper, and garlic salt. Mix thoroughly.

- Drain and mash artichokes; place in bottom of buttered 2-quart casserole. Cover with spinach mixture. Sprinkle generously with Parmesan cheese and dot with butter. Bake 30 to 40 minutes. Serves 8 to 10.

Mrs. Jack W. Hoelscher (Barbara)

Baked Herb Tomatoes

2 cups canned tomatoes, undrained
½ tablespoon sugar
1 teaspoon salt
¼ teaspoon rosemary
1 cup poultry stuffing
  (reserve ¼ cup for topping)

1 small onion, finely chopped
¼ teaspoon oregano
Butter

- Preheat oven to 350 degrees.

- Combine tomatoes, sugar, salt, rosemary, poultry stuffing, onion, and oregano. Pour into greased 1-quart casserole.

- Sprinkle with ¼ cup poultry stuffing and dot with butter. Bake 45 minutes. Serves 4.

Mrs. James B. Cochran (Linda)

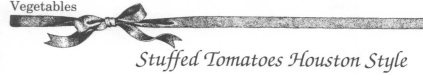

Stuffed Tomatoes Houston Style

10 ripe medium tomatoes
1 bunch green onions with tops,
   chopped
2 garlic cloves, crushed
¼ cup butter
¼ cup olive oil
1 tablespoon oregano
½ teaspoon red pepper

½ teaspoon basil
2 bay leaves
½ teaspoon thyme
2 (3-ounce) cans chopped
   mushrooms, undrained
Salt to taste
1 cup Italian seasoned breadcrumbs
½ cup grated Parmesan cheese

• Preheat oven to 350 degrees.

• Cut stem end off tomatoes; scoop out pulp with spoon, chop and reserve. Turn shells upside down to drain.

• Sauté onions and garlic in butter and oil until soft; add oregano, red pepper, basil, bay leaves, thyme, and mushrooms with liquid. Cook 5 minutes.

• Add tomato pulp and salt to taste. Simmer 20 to 30 minutes; remove bay leaves. Add breadcrumbs and cheese. Stir well.

• Stuff mixture into shells. Sprinkle with extra Parmesan cheese. Bake 20 to 30 minutes. Serves 10.

Mrs. Phillip Sherman, Jr. (Sandy)

Steamed Zucchini

4 tablespoons margarine
5 or 6 small zucchini, sliced
1 medium onion, sliced

1 (7-ounce) package Italian dressing
   mix

• Melt margarine in skillet. Add sliced zucchini and onion. Sprinkle dressing mix on top.

• Cover and cook slowly 15 to 20 minutes until done, stirring once or twice. Serves 6 to 8.

Mrs. Percy A. Bennett, Jr. (Dot)

Use twice the amount of fresh herbs when substituting for dried herbs.

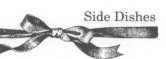

David's Hollandaise Sauce

4 egg yolks
2 tablespoons fresh lemon juice

1 cup margarine

- In saucepan, beat egg yolks and stir in lemon juice. Add margarine.

- Cook very slowly over low heat, stirring constantly with wire whisk until margarine melts and sauce thickens. Makes 1 cup.

Mrs. David R. Libby (Donna)

Baked Apricots

2 (28-ounce) cans apricots, drained
½ (1-pound) box light brown sugar
½ (12-ounce) box round buttery crackers, crushed in blender

Butter

- Preheat oven to 300 degrees.

- Place apricots in lightly greased 3-quart casserole.

- Cover with light brown sugar. Top with cracker crumbs. Dot with butter. Bake 1 hour. Serves 10 to 12.

Great accompaniment with meat or poultry.

Mrs. David B. Fox (Sallie)

Baked Bananas

4 to 6 bananas, peeled and sliced lengthwise
1 (8-ounce) jar orange marmalade

1 (2-ounce) package slivered almonds

- Preheat oven to 350 degrees.

- Place banana halves in well buttered baking dish. Coat top of bananas with marmalade. Sprinkle with almonds.

- Bake 10 minutes or until bubbly. Serves 6.

Great brunch side dish!

Mrs. William O. Coley, Jr. (Fran)

Fresh Cranberry Sauce

3¼ cups sugar
2 cups water
½ cup orange juice

2 (12-ounce) packages cranberries
1 tablespoon grated orange rind

- In a 4 to 8-quart container combine sugar, water, and orange juice. Bring to boil over low heat and simmer 5 to 10 minutes, or until sugar is dissolved.

- Add rinsed cranberries and cook over moderately high heat 4 to 5 minutes, or until berries have popped. Stir in orange rind and cool. Refrigerate. Will keep 2 weeks. Makes 1½ quarts.

Our whole family gathers to see and hear the cranberries pop at Thanksgiving and Christmas. Wonderful holiday treat to share!

Mrs. David R. Libby (Donna)

Honey Baked Fruit

1 (16-ounce) can apricots
1 (16-ounce) can pears
1 (16-ounce) can black cherries,
   pitted
1 (16-ounce) can pineapple chunks
1 cup applesauce

1 (10-ounce) package frozen
   raspberries
¼ cup honey
2 tablespoons frozen orange juice
   concentrate

- Preheat oven to 350 degrees.

- Drain fruit and arrange in 3-quart casserole.

- Mix honey and orange juice and pour over top.

- Bake 20 minutes. Serves 8 to 10.

Mrs. Warren L. Lesmeister (Carol)

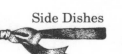

Hot Fruit Compote

12 dried macaroons, crumbled and divided
4 cups canned fruit, well drained (peaches, pears, apricots, pineapple, cherries)

½ cup toasted slivered almonds or pecans
½ cup brown sugar
½ cup cooking sherry
¼ cup melted butter

- Preheat oven to 350 degrees.

- Butter 2½-quart casserole. Cover bottom with ½ crumbled macaroons.

- In layers, arrange fruit, finishing with macaroons. Sprinkle with almonds, brown sugar and sherry.

- Bake uncovered 30 minutes. Remove from oven and drizzle melted butter over top. Serves 8 to 10. Serve hot.

Excellent accompaniment for ham.

Mrs. Joe Hall Morris (Adair)

Hot Gingered Fruit

1 (16-ounce) can cling peach halves
1 (16-ounce) can whole pitted apricots
1 (16-ounce) can pineapple slices
1 (16-ounce) can pear halves

1 (6-ounce) jar maraschino cherries
¼ cup margarine
½ teaspoon ginger
¾ cup light brown sugar

- Preheat oven to 325 degrees.

- Drain all fruit, reserving 2 tablespoons pineapple syrup. Dry fruit well on paper towels. Arrange in 2-quart casserole; place cherries on top.

- Melt margarine with ginger in small pan. Stir in pineapple syrup and sugar. Heat until sugar melts.

- Pour over fruit and bake 40 minutes. Serves 10 to 12.

Variation: Substitute 1½ teaspoons curry powder for ginger.

Mrs. C. Dale Moody, Jr. (Doris)

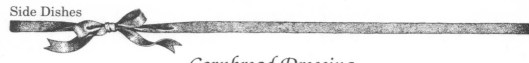

Cornbread Dressing

2 medium onions, chopped
1 small bunch celery with leaves,
   chopped
½ bunch parsley, chopped
½ cup butter
4 teaspoons poultry seasoning
1 teaspoon salt

¼ teaspoon pepper
1 teaspoon sage
1 10-inch skillet cornbread
4 to 5 leftover biscuits or slices
   white bread
4 to 6 cups turkey or chicken broth

- Preheat oven to 400 degrees.

- Sauté onion, celery, and parsley in butter until tender.

- Combine seasonings and coarsely crumbled bread. Add onion mixture and enough broth to make dressing moist. Bake in greased 3-quart casserole for 25 minutes. Serves 12 to 15.

*Chopped pecans, sautéed mushrooms, or
cooked pork sausage may be added to dressing if desired.*

Mrs. John Mallett Barron (Doy)

Oyster Casserole

1 pint oysters
2 cups cracker crumbs
½ cup butter
½ teaspoon salt

Dash pepper
¾ cup half-and-half
¼ cup oyster liquid
½ teaspoon Worcestershire sauce

- Preheat oven to 350 degrees.

- Drain oysters and reserve liquid. Combine crumbs, butter, and salt.

- In 1½-quart greased casserole, layer ⅓ cracker crumb mixture and ½ of oysters sprinkled with pepper; repeat, then combine half-and-half, oyster liquid, and Worcestershire and pour over layers. Top with remaining ⅓ cracker crumbs.

- Bake 40 minutes. Serves 8.

Wonderful holiday accompaniment for turkey and dressing.

Mrs. Charles E. Harbison (Betty)

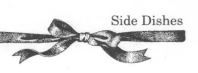

Pear Chutney

4½ pounds ripe pears
1 large green bell pepper
1½ cups seedless raisins
1 cup chopped crystallized ginger
4 cups sugar
3 cups vinegar
1 cup water

½ teaspoon salt
6 bay leaves
¼ teaspoon ground cloves
¼ teaspoon allspice
¼ teaspoon nutmeg
½ teaspoon cinnamon
½ cup bottled liquid pectin

- Pare, core, and slice pears. Chop bell pepper.

- In saucepan, mix all ingredients except pectin.

- Simmer until pears are tender and mixture is thick, about 2 hours. Remove bay leaves and add pectin. Boil 1 minute. Pour into jars and seal. Yields 2 to 3 quarts.

Perfect holiday gift.

Mrs. James F. Bennett, Jr. (Ann)

Pickled Pears

2 cups cider vinegar
2 cups sugar
2 tablespoons whole pickling spice

2 cups apple juice
12 large, very firm pears, halved

- In saucepan, combine vinegar, sugar, spice, and apple juice. Bring to boil. Add pears and simmer until just tender, but still hold shape.

- Place pears in sterilized jars. Add juice to cover. (Pears above juice will turn brown.) Refrigerate. Makes 24 halves.

This fills the house with a wonderful aroma! Makes a nice Christmas gift.

Mrs. Ernest H. Sigman, Jr. (Doris)

Betty's Spiced Peaches

1 (28-ounce) can peach halves
1 (3-inch) stick cinnamon
1 teaspoon whole cloves

1 teaspoon allspice
¼ cup white vinegar

- Drain syrup from peaches into saucepan. Add spices and vinegar. Simmer 5 minutes. Pour over peaches and refrigerate overnight.

- Sauce can be reused. Add more drained peaches and chill.

Mrs. J. Howard McClain (Virginia)

Pineapple Cheese Casserole

2 eggs
⅓ cup sugar
Dash salt
2 tablespoons flour
1 (20-ounce) can pineapple chunks,
  drained and juice reserved

1½ cups Velveeta cheese, cut into
  small chunks
1 (16-ounce) package marshmallows

- Preheat oven to 350 degrees.

- Beat eggs in saucepan. Add sugar, salt, flour, and juice from pineapple. Cook until thick, stirring constantly.

- Put cheese and pineapple in 2-quart greased Pyrex dish. Cover with sauce and top with marshmallows. Bake 20 to 25 minutes. Serves 6 to 8.

Great side dish with ham or turkey.

Mrs. Thad L. Morris (Barbara)

Pickled Okra

1 to 2 pounds of fresh okra
Ice water
Garlic cloves

Dill leaves
Red pepper strips

- Wash and trim okra; soak in ice water for 24 hours. Sterilize jars and in each jar place clove of garlic, clump of dill and ½x2-inch strip red pepper. Rinse okra and pack in jars alternating the ends. Pour in hot pickling solution until jar is full. Let jars stand for an hour until solution stops bubbling. Refill jars to brim again and screw on cap tightly.

Pickling Solution:
1 quart vinegar
2 quarts water

1 scant cup salt
1 pea-sized piece of alum

- Bring ingredients to boil. Stir well and keep at low boil 10 to 15 minutes. Solution must be hot when used. Excess may be kept and used later but must be reheated.

Mrs. James N. McLaughlin (Gwenice)

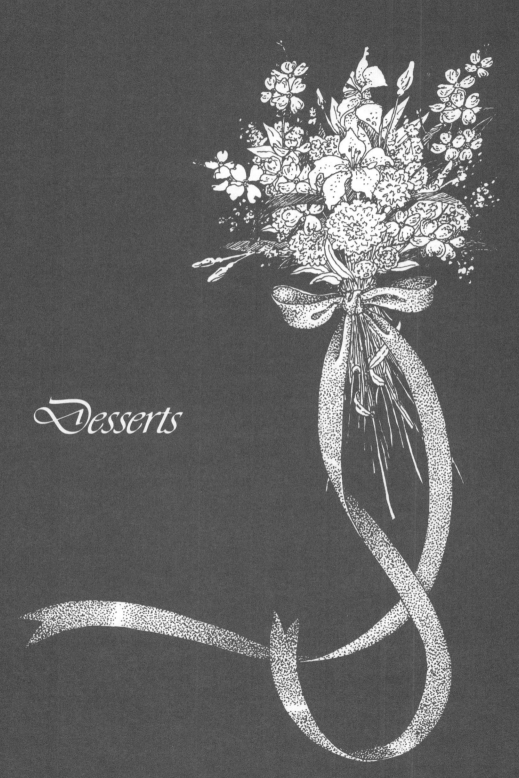

Desserts

Apple Pie

**1 (10-inch) pie crust, unbaked
(see pumpkin pie in index)**

- Preheat oven to 375 degrees.
- Prick crust with fork several times to keep from bubbling. Bake 8 minutes.

Topping:
¼ **cup butter, melted**   ½ **cup flour**
¼ **cup sugar**   ½ **cup shredded cheddar cheese**

- Mix ingredients together until crumbly; set aside.

Filling:
½ **cup white sugar**   **6 cups peeled, thinly sliced tart**
½ **cup light brown sugar**   **cooking apples**
2 tablespoons flour   **1 tablespoon lemon juice**
1 teaspoon cinnamon   **1 tablespoon sherry**
¼ **teaspoon nutmeg**

- Preheat oven to 400 degrees.
- Mix together sugars, flour, cinnamon, and nutmeg. Coat sliced apples.
- Add lemon juice and sherry; toss apple mixture. Put in pie crust, sprinkle topping mixture over apples, and bake 15 minutes.
- Turn oven to 350 degrees and bake 35 to 45 minutes until bubbly in center and lightly brown. Serves 8.

Mrs. P. D. Miller, Jr. (Greene)

*F*or tender, flaky pastry, chill all ingredients before combining, handle as little as possible, and add flour sparingly when rolling.

*R*oll pie crust in waxed paper. Turn upside down over pie plate, roll off waxed paper.

*T*o prevent apples from turning brown while peeling, slice into a bowl of cold, slightly salted water.

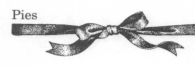

Banana Cream Pie

1 cup sugar	1 teaspoon vanilla
3 tablespoons cornstarch	3 bananas, sliced
¼ teaspoon salt	1 (9-inch) pie shell, baked and
2 cups milk	cooled
3 egg yolks, slightly beaten	1 cup whipping cream, whipped

- Combine sugar, cornstarch, salt, and milk in saucepan. Cook and stir over medium heat until mixture boils and thickens. Cook 2 more minutes. Remove from heat.

- Stir small amount hot mixture into yolks; return to hot mixture and cook 2 minutes, stirring constantly. Remove from heat; add vanilla and cool to room temperature.

- Slice 3 bananas into pie shell. Top with filling and spread whipped cream on top. Refrigerate. Serves 6.

Mrs. David R. Libby (Donna)

Southern Chess Pie

3 eggs, beaten	6 tablespoons buttermilk
1½ cups sugar	6 tablespoons butter, melted
1 teaspoon vanilla	1 (9-inch) pie shell, unbaked

- Preheat oven to 350 degrees.

- Mix first 5 ingredients together and pour into pie shell.

- Bake 30 minutes, then 10 minutes at 300 degrees or until pie is set. Serves 6 to 8.

Freezes well.

Mrs. John Mallett Barron (Doy)

Cream is easiest to whip when chilled. Also chill bowl and beaters.

Cocoa Cream Pie

1 cup sugar
⅓ cup cocoa
¼ cup flour
½ teaspoon salt
3 eggs
¼ cup butter, melted

¾ cup dark corn syrup
¾ cup evaporated milk
1 teaspoon vanilla
1 cup pecan halves
1 (9-inch) pie shell, unbaked
Whipped cream

- Preheat oven to 425 degrees.

- Sift together sugar, cocoa, flour, and salt. Set aside.

- Beat eggs well and blend with melted butter, syrup, milk, and vanilla. Add dry ingredients to egg mixture and blend well.

- Stir in pecans and pour into pie crust. Pecans will rise to top. Bake 10 minutes. Lower heat to 325 degrees and bake 40 minutes.

- Cool before serving. Top with whipped cream. Serves 6.

Mrs. Danny Weiss (Saralyn)

Chocolate Fudge Pie

2 cups sugar
2 tablespoons flour
¼ cup cocoa
⅛ teaspoon salt
4 eggs

⅔ cup butter or margarine, melted
3 teaspoons vanilla
2 (9-inch) pie shells, unbaked
Whipped cream or peppermint ice cream

- Preheat oven to 350 degrees.

- Mix sugar, flour, cocoa, and salt; add beaten eggs, butter, and vanilla.

- Pour into pie shells and bake 30 minutes. Garnish with whipped cream or ice cream.

Mrs. Carl L. Sebelius, Jr. (Judy)

A pinch of salt added to heavy cream will make it whip faster.

Fudge Pie

2 (1-ounce) squares unsweetened chocolate
½ cup margarine
1 cup sugar

¼ cup flour
2 eggs, beaten
½ teaspoon vanilla

- Preheat oven to 350 degrees.

- Melt chocolate and margarine.

- Combine sugar and flour and stir in chocolate mixture. Add eggs and vanilla, stirring until well mixed. Pour into greased 9-inch pie plate and bake 25 minutes. Serve hot with ice cream. Serves 6 to 8.

A great last minute dessert!

Dr. David R. Libby

Angel Chocolate Pie

Meringue Crust:
2 egg whites
½ cup sugar
⅛ teaspoon cream of tartar

⅛ teaspoon salt
½ cup chopped pecans

- Preheat oven to 275 degrees.

- Beat egg whites until stiff; add sugar, cream of tartar, and salt. Fold in pecans. Bake in well greased 9-inch pie pan 1 hour. Turn oven off, leave meringue in unopened oven approximately 2 hours.

Filling:
1 cup whipping cream
4 ounces semi-sweet chocolate

3 tablespoons water
1 tablespoon brandy

- Whip cream. Melt chocolate in water and cool. Add brandy to cooled chocolate and fold into cream. Pour into shell and refrigerate. Serves 6.

Mrs. Richard J. Reynolds (Anne)

French Silk Chocolate Pie

Meringue Crust:

2 egg whites
⅛ teaspoon salt
⅛ teaspoon cream of tartar

½ cup sugar
½ cup chopped pecans
½ teaspoon vanilla

- Preheat oven to 300 degrees.

- Beat egg whites with salt and cream of tartar until foamy. Add sugar, 1 tablespoon at a time, beating until very stiff peaks hold.

- Fold in pecans and vanilla. Spread in 9-inch greased pie pan. Bake 50 to 55 minutes. Cool.

Filling:

½ cup margarine
¾ cup sugar
1½ squares unsweetened chocolate, melted and cooled

1 teaspoon vanilla
2 egg yolks
2 eggs

- Cream margarine and add sugar gradually. Blend in melted chocolate and vanilla.

- Add 2 egg yolks and 2 eggs, one at a time, beating 5 minutes after each addition. Pour into meringue shell and refrigerate. Serves 6.

Serve topped with whipped cream and finely chopped pecans.

Mrs. A. Joe Fuson (Jean)

Chocolate Chess Pie

3 tablespoons cocoa
1½ cups sugar
2 eggs
1 (5-ounce) can evaporated milk

¼ cup butter, softened
1 teaspoon vanilla
1 (8-inch) pie shell, unbaked

- Preheat oven to 400 degrees.

- Mix cocoa and sugar. Add eggs, milk, butter, and vanilla. Pour into pie shell. Bake 15 minutes, reduce oven temperature to 250 degrees and continue baking 30 minutes.

Mrs. Richard C. Harris (Beverly)
Mrs. George H. Bouldien (Judy)

Delta Chocolate Pie

1 cup sugar
½ cup flour
2 eggs
½ cup margarine, melted
1 cup chopped pecans

1 cup chocolate chips
1 teaspoon vanilla
1 (9-inch) pie shell,
  unbaked

- Preheat oven to 350 degrees.

- Mix sugar and flour. Add eggs and margarine. Mix well.

- Add nuts, chocolate chips, and vanilla. Pour into pie shell and bake 30 to 40 minutes. Serves 6 to 8.

Mrs. Robert Hatch (Nat)
Mrs. Robert L. Gardino (Ann)

"Watch Your Weight" Chocolate Cream Pie

6 tablespoons crunchy peanut
  butter
2 tablespoons honey
1½ cups Rice Krispies
1 banana

1 (3¾-ounce) box sugar-free
  chocolate pudding
2 cups skim milk
1 cup Cool Whip

- Mix well the peanut butter, honey, and Rice Krispies. Press in 9-inch pie pan and slice banana over crust.

- Mix chocolate pudding with milk. Pour over banana slices and chill 30 minutes. Spread Cool Whip over top.

Mrs. J. B. Edmonds (Jeanne)

Be certain a meringue topping on a pie touches the edge of the crust so that it will not shrink from the sides.

Impossible Coconut Pie

4 eggs
2 cups sugar
½ cup flour
½ teaspoon baking powder
⅛ teaspoon salt

2 cups milk
½ cup butter, melted
1 teaspoon vanilla
1 cup flaked coconut

- Preheat oven to 350 degrees.

- Beat eggs and add sugar.

- Sift together flour, baking powder, and salt; add to egg mixture, mixing well.

- Add milk gradually, stirring until well blended. Stir in butter, vanilla and coconut.

- Pour into lightly greased 13x9x2-inch pan or two 8-inch pie pans. Bake 30 minutes or until set. Serves 8 to 10.

This pie makes its own crust as it bakes.

Mrs. Thad L. Morris (Barbara)

Howard McClain's Easy Pie

3 eggs
1 cup sugar
¼ cup margarine, melted
¼ cup buttermilk

1⅓ cups flaked coconut
1 teaspoon vanilla
1 (9-inch) pie shell, unbaked

- Preheat oven to 375 degrees.

- Beat eggs slightly; add remaining ingredients and mix well. Pour into pie shell.

- Bake 10 minutes. Lower heat to 300 degrees and bake about 35 minutes or until golden brown. Serves 6.

Mrs. Warren L. Lesmeister (Carol)

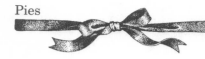

Lemonade Pie

1 (6-ounce) can frozen lemonade
  concentrate
1 (4-ounce) carton whipped topping

1 (14-ounce) can sweetened
  condensed milk
1 (9-inch) graham cracker crust

- Thaw lemonade. Combine lemonade, topping, and condensed milk. Beat thoroughly.

- Pour into pie crust and chill. Serves 6.

Notice: No eggs for cholesterol watchers!

Mrs. John Mallett Barron (Doy)
Mrs. Joe L. Cannon (Nell)

Colonial Pecan Pie

Basic Pie Crust (Food Processor):
1½ cups flour
½ teaspoon salt
1 tablespoon shortening
7 tablespoons chilled butter, cut
  into chunks

4 tablespoons ice water
1 teaspoon white vinegar

- Blend first 4 ingredients in food processor until crumbly. Add remaining ingredients and blend a few seconds until dough begins to form a ball. Divide and chill 1 to 2 hours.

- Roll out on floured board. Makes two 8-inch crusts.

Filling:
3 eggs
6 tablespoons sugar
3 tablespoons firmly packed brown
  sugar
2 level teaspoons flour
3 tablespoons butter, melted

1 cup light corn syrup
⅛ teaspoon salt
1 teaspoon vanilla
1 cup coarsely chopped pecans
1 (9-inch) deep dish pie crust,
  unbaked

- Preheat oven to 400 degrees.

- Beat eggs slightly; add next seven ingredients and mix well. Stir in pecans. Pour into crust. Bake 15 minutes. Reduce heat to 350 degrees and bake about 35 minutes until pie is firm. Serves 6 to 8.

Mrs. James F. Bennett, Jr. (Ann)
Mrs. J. Roy Bourgoyne (Helen Ruth)

Kahlúa Pecan Pie

¼ cup butter
¾ cup sugar
1 teaspoon vanilla
2 tablespoons flour
3 eggs
½ cup Kahlúa

½ cup dark corn syrup
¾ cup evaporated milk
1 (10-inch) pie shell, chilled
1 cup pecan halves
Whipped cream, optional

- Preheat oven to 400 degrees.

- Cream butter, sugar, vanilla, and flour. Beat in eggs, one at a time. Stir in Kahlúa, corn syrup, evaporated milk, and pecans.

- Pour into pie shell and bake 10 minutes. Reduce heat to 325 degrees and bake about 40 minutes or until firm.

- Chill 8 hours or overnight. When ready to serve, garnish with whipped cream and pecan halves if desired. Serves 8 to 10.

Mrs. Morris L. Robbins (Laura Dee)

Pecan Tarts

Dough:
1 (3-ounce) package cream cheese, softened
½ cup butter, softened

1 cup flour
Dash salt

- Combine all ingredients until well blended. Refrigerate 1 hour. Pinch dough into small balls. Place each ball into miniature muffin tins and press to form shells.

Filling:
1 egg
¾ cup light brown sugar
1 tablespoon soft butter

1 teaspoon vanilla
Dash salt
2 cups chopped pecans

- Preheat oven to 350 degrees.

- Beat together egg, brown sugar, butter, vanilla, and salt. Stir in pecans. Pour into pie shells in muffin tins.

- Bake 15 to 20 minutes until lightly brown. Cool before removing from tins. Makes 36.

Mrs. Larry Weiss (Susan)

Southern Peach Pie

5 cups sliced fresh peaches
1 (9-inch) pie shell, unbaked
⅓ cup margarine, melted
1 cup sugar

⅓ cup flour
1 egg, slightly beaten
Ice cream, optional

• Preheat oven to 350 degrees.

• Place peaches in pie shell. Combine remaining ingredients and pour over peaches. Bake 1 hour and 10 minutes. Top with ice cream, if desired. Serves 6.

Mrs. James R. Wyatt (Mary Kate)

Pineapple Cream Cheese Pie

⅓ cup sugar
1 tablespoon cornstarch
1 (9-ounce) can crushed pineapple, undrained
1 (8-ounce) package cream cheese, softened
½ cup sugar

½ teaspoon salt
2 eggs
½ cup milk
½ teaspoon vanilla
1 (9-inch) pie shell, unbaked
¼ cup chopped pecans

• Preheat oven to 400 degrees.

• Blend ⅓ cup sugar with cornstarch and add pineapple. Cook, stirring constantly, until mixture is thick and clear. Cool.

• Blend cream cheese with ½ cup sugar and salt. Add eggs, one at a time, stirring well after each. Blend in milk and vanilla.

• Spread the cooled pineapple mixture over bottom of pie shell. Pour in cream cheese mixture and sprinkle with chopped pecans.

• Bake 10 minutes. Reduce temperature to 325 degrees and bake 50 minutes. Cool before serving.

Mrs. James L. Wiygul (Lou)

Pumpkin Pie

Crust:

2 cups flour
1 teaspoon salt

⅔ cup shortening
⅓ cup ice water

- Preheat oven to 375 degrees.

- Mix flour and salt; cut in shortening. Add ice water and mix well with fork until dough forms. Chill. Roll into two 9-inch pie crusts. Bake 8 minutes.

Filling:

2 eggs, beaten
2 cups pumpkin
1½ cups sugar
2 cups half-and-half
½ teaspoon salt

1 teaspoon ginger
1 teaspoon cinnamon
½ teaspoon nutmeg
2 tablespoons butter, melted

- Preheat oven to 400 degrees.

- Beat eggs, add pumpkin, sugar, half-and-half, salt, spices, and melted butter. Mix in blender until smooth. Pour into crusts. Bake 15 minutes. Turn oven to 350 degrees and bake 45 minutes. Makes two 9-inch pies.

Fresh steamed pumpkin makes a better pie.

Mrs. P. D. Miller, Jr. (Greene)

Soda Cracker Pie

3 egg whites
½ teaspoon baking powder
1 cup sugar
1 cup chopped pecans

14 soda crackers, crushed
1 cup whipping cream, whipped
¼ teaspoon vanilla

- Preheat oven to 350 degrees.

- Beat egg whites until peaks form. Add baking powder and gradually add sugar while beating. Fold in nuts and crackers. Pour into greased 9-inch pie plate. Bake 30 minutes.

- Cool. Before serving, top with whipped cream flavored with vanilla. Chill. Serves 6.

Mrs. H. Ray Manning (Rose Marie)

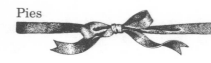

Sherry Pie

4 tablespoons water
1 envelope unflavored gelatin
¼ teaspoon salt
1 cup milk
½ cup sugar
3 egg yolks, beaten

3 egg whites, stiffly beaten
⅛ teaspoon nutmeg
½ cup sherry
1 cup whipping cream, whipped
1 (9-inch) pastry or graham cracker
    crumb pie shell, baked

• In small bowl combine water, gelatin, and salt. Set aside.

• In double boiler combine milk, sugar, and egg yolks. Mix together thoroughly; cook mixture until it coats spoon. Add dissolved gelatin to hot mixture; stir until dissolved. Let mixture cool.

• Fold in egg whites, nutmeg, sherry, and whipped cream. Put mixture into pie shell. Chill overnight.

Garnish with grated chocolate.

Mrs. Thad L. Morris (Barbara)

Fresh Strawberry Pie

½ cup fresh lemon juice
1 (14-ounce) can sweetened
    condensed milk
1 (8-ounce) carton whipped topping

1 quart fresh strawberries, washed
    and halved
1 (10-inch) graham cracker pie
    shell, or 2 (8-inch) shells

• Combine lemon juice and condensed milk and mix well. Fold in whipped topping and strawberries.

• Pour into pie shell and refrigerate 2 hours. Serves 8 to 10.

May omit strawberries and use filling as a light lemon dessert served in sherbets, topped with sliced kiwi fruit.

Mrs. David R. Libby (Donna)

Separate yolks and whites while eggs are cold for easier separation.

Fresh Apple Cake

Cake:

1½ cups salad oil
2 cups sugar
3 eggs
2 teaspoons vanilla
3 cups flour

1 teaspoon baking soda
½ teaspoon salt
1 cup chopped pecans or walnuts
3 cups peeled, chopped apples

- Preheat oven to 350 degrees.

- Mix first four ingredients. Add sifted flour, soda, and salt. Fold in nuts and apples. Pour into well greased 10-inch fluted tube pan; bake 1 hour. Remove cake from pan while still warm.

Frosting:

1 cup brown sugar
½ cup evaporated milk

1 cup confectioners' sugar

- Bring brown sugar and evaporated milk to a boil and boil 2 minutes. Blend in confectioners' sugar. Beat until smooth and pour over cake.

Mrs. James F. Bennett, Jr. (Ann)

Apple-Butterscotch Sheet Cake

2 cups sugar
2 eggs
1 scant cup oil
2½ cups flour
2 teaspoons baking soda
1 teaspoon salt

¾ teaspoon cinnamon
3 tart apples, diced
1 cup chopped nuts
1 (12-ounce) package butterscotch morsels, divided

- Preheat oven to 325 degrees.

- Mix sugar, eggs, and oil. Sift in flour, soda, salt, and cinnamon. Mix well.

- Add apples, nuts, and half of butterscotch morsels.

- Pour into greased and floured 15x10x1-inch jelly-roll pan. Sprinkle remaining morsels over batter. Bake 1 hour or until brown.

Mrs. James B. Cochran (Linda)

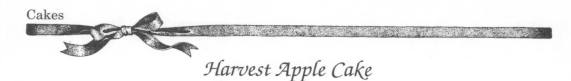

Harvest Apple Cake

1 egg
1 cup sugar
⅔ scant cup vegetable oil
1½ cups flour
1 teaspoon baking soda

Dash salt
2 cups chopped apples
1 cup chopped pecans
1 teaspoon vanilla

- Preheat oven to 350 degrees.

- Beat egg; add remaining ingredients.

- Bake in greased and floured 8-inch square baking pan 30 minutes or longer.

Mrs. Charles E. Wilkinson (Jo Anne)

Black Russian Cake

Cake:
1 box dark chocolate cake mix
1 cup vegetable oil
1 (3½-ounce) package instant
   chocolate pudding

4 eggs
¾ cup strong coffee
½ cup crème de cacao
¼ cup Kahlúa

- Preheat oven to 350 degrees.

- Combine all ingredients and beat 4 minutes at medium speed. Pour into well greased 10-inch tube pan. Bake 45 to 50 minutes. Remove from pan and punch holes in top.

Topping:
1 cup confectioners' sugar, sifted
2 tablespoons strong coffee

2 tablespoons Kahlúa
2 tablespoons crème de cacao

- Combine ingredients and mix well. Spoon over warm cake.

Mrs. Joe Hall Morris (Adair)

Cooked frostings do not freeze well.

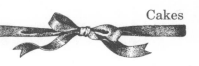

Carrot Cake

Cake:

4 eggs
2 cups sugar
1¼ cups vegetable oil
2 cups flour
2 teaspoons baking powder

2 teaspoons baking soda
2 teaspoons cinnamon
3 cups finely grated carrots
½ cup chopped pecans

- Preheat oven to 325 degrees.

- Beat eggs; add sugar and oil. Sift dry ingredients and add. Stir in carrots and pecans.

- Bake in greased and floured 13x9x2-inch pan 40 minutes.

Frosting:

1 (8-ounce) package cream cheese
½ cup margarine
1 teaspoon vanilla

1 (16-ounce) box confectioners' sugar

- Cream all ingredients and spread on cooled cake.

Mrs. Jack C. Brooks (Betty Lou)

Richglen's Cheddar Cheesecake with Strawberries

1¼ cups vanilla wafer crumbs
2 tablespoons butter or margarine, melted
2 (8-ounce) packages cream cheese, softened
½ cup shredded sharp cheddar cheese
¾ cup sugar

3 eggs
½ teaspoon grated orange peel
¼ teaspoon grated lemon peel
2 tablespoons flour
1 cup whipping cream, divided
1 pint fresh strawberries
Light corn syrup

- Preheat oven to 350 degrees.

- Mix crumbs with butter; press over bottom of 9-inch springform pan. Bake 5 minutes.

- Combine the cheeses and sugar; beat until fluffy. Beat in eggs, one at a time. Blend in peels, flour, and ½ cup of cream. Pour over crumb crust and bake 40 minutes, until set in center. Cool on rack.

- Arrange whole strawberries on top of cake. Brush with corn syrup.

- Whip remaining cream until stiff; using a pastry tube, pipe in border around the strawberries.

Mrs. James R. Ross (Lucy)

Cocoa Cheesecake

Crust:
⅓ cup butter, melted
2 tablespoons sugar

1½ cups zwieback crumbs (18
   pieces)

• Combine crust ingredients and press mixture on bottom and 1½ to 2-inches up the side of 8-inch springform pan and refrigerate.

Filling:
2 (8-ounce) packages cream cheese,
   softened
1¼ cups sugar

⅓ cup cocoa
1 teaspoon vanilla
2 eggs

• Preheat oven to 375 degrees.

• Beat cream cheese until smooth; add remaining ingredients. Pour into prepared crust and bake 25 minutes.

Topping:
1 cup sour cream

½ teaspoon vanilla

• Combine sour cream and vanilla. Spread over top of baked filling and return to oven; bake 10 minutes.

• Cool on wire rack; chill thoroughly.

Garnish:
½ cup whipping cream, whipped

1 tablespoon grated semi-sweet
   chocolate

Mrs. David Neal (Cissie)

The secret to making successful chocolate curls is having the chocolate bar at the proper temperature, slightly warm, but still firm. Chocolate curls can be refrigerated and stored for later use.

Favorite Cheesecake

Crust:
1½ cups graham cracker crumbs   ½ cup butter, melted
½ cup sugar

- Mix crust ingredients and pat in bottom of 10-inch tube pan. Grease side of pan with small amount of butter and set aside.

Filling:
3 (8-ounce) packages cream cheese   1½ cups sugar
5 eggs   2 teaspoons vanilla

Topping:
3 cups sour cream   1 cup sugar
2 teaspoons vanilla

- Preheat oven to 300 degrees.

- Beat cream cheese until soft; add one egg at a time, beating well. Add sugar slowly, beating well. Add vanilla and pour into crust.

- Bake 1 hour. Remove from oven and top with combined topping ingredients. Return to oven 15 minutes. Remove from oven and cool 30 minutes.

- Refrigerate at least 6 hours. Lift tube and slice to serve.

Mrs. Nathan R. Walley (Donna)

Don't overcook or your cheesecake will be dry!

Mini Cheesecakes

3 (8-ounce) packages cream cheese,
  softened
1 cup sugar

5 eggs
½ teaspoon vanilla

- Preheat oven to 300 degrees.

- Mix all ingredients until there are no lumps.

- Fill midget foil baking cups ¾ full on cookie sheet and bake 30 to 40 minutes. Cool.

Topping:
1 cup sour cream
¼ cup sugar

½ teaspoon vanilla
Strawberry preserves

- Combine sour cream, sugar, and vanilla; put a small amount on top of each cake. Dot with strawberry preserves. Bake 5 minutes. Freezes well. Yields 48.

Mrs. Jack W. Hoelscher (Barbara)

Chocolate Marshmallow Cake

¾ cup margarine
2 cups sugar
3½ tablespoons cocoa
3 eggs
2 cups self-rising flour

1 teaspoon vanilla
1½ cups chopped pecans
1 (6¼-ounce) package miniature
  marshmallows

- Preheat oven to 325 degrees.

- Cream margarine and sugar. Add cocoa, eggs, flour, and vanilla; mix well. Stir in pecans. Pour into greased 13x9x2-inch baking pan.

- Bake 40 minutes. When done, spread marshmallows on top and melt in oven 5 minutes. Cool 30 minutes.

Topping:
¾ cup margarine, melted
1 (16-ounce) box confectioners'
  sugar

4½ tablespoons cocoa
½ cup evaporated milk
1 teaspoon vanilla

- Mix topping ingredients and pour over cake. Allow to set overnight.

Mrs. James F. Bennett, Jr. (Ann)

Chocolate Fudge Oreo Sundae Cake

Crust:
1 pound oreo cookies, crushed   **½ cup margarine, melted**

• Mix oreos and margarine and press into 13x9x2-inch pan.

Filling:
½ gallon chocolate chip or fudge
  ripple ice cream, softened

• Spread ice cream over crust and freeze.

Sauce:
¾ cup chocolate morsels   **1 (5-ounce) can evaporated milk**
½ cup margarine   **2 cups confectioners' sugar**

• Combine ingredients in saucepan and boil 8 minutes.

• Pour over ice cream and serve immediately or freeze. Serves 16.

*May slice 2 to 3 bananas, nuts, and coconut
onto crust before spreading ice cream.*

Mrs. Robert L. Parrish. Jr. (Kaye)

Best Ever Chocolate Cake

1 (18.25-ounce) Duncan Hines   **½ cup oil**
  Devil's Food cake mix   **½ cup cold coffee**
1 (3½-ounce) box instant chocolate   **1 cup sour cream**
  pudding   **1 (12-ounce) package chocolate**
4 eggs   **morsels**

• Preheat oven to 350 degrees.

• Mix well all ingredients, except chocolate morsels. After mixing, gently fold morsels into batter.

• Pour into 10-inch well greased bundt pan and bake 50 minutes. Ice with favorite icing, or sprinkle with confectioners' sugar.

Mrs. Norman Towbin (Barbara)

Chocolate Chip Date Cake

Topping:
½ cup brown sugar   ½ cup chopped pecans
1 (6-ounce) package chocolate chips

• Combine topping ingredients and set aside.

Cake:
1½ cups boiling water   2 eggs
1 (8-ounce) package dates, chopped   1½ cups flour, sifted
1 teaspoon baking soda   1 teaspoon vanilla
1 cup margarine   ⅛ teaspoon salt
1 cup sugar   1 cup whipping cream, whipped

• Preheat oven to 350 degrees.

• Combine water, dates, and soda in large bowl and let stand until cool.

• Cream margarine and sugar. Add eggs, flour, vanilla, and salt. Add date mixture.

• Pour into greased 13x9x2-inch baking pan. Sprinkle with topping. Bake 45 minutes. Serves 12 to 15.

• When ready to serve top with whipped cream.

Mrs. Joseph W. Graham (Billie Jean)

For chocolate cakes, dust pan with cocoa instead of flour for a more attractive and tastier concoction.

Chocolate Sheet Cake

2 cups flour
2 cups sugar
1 teaspoon cinnamon
1 teaspoon baking soda
½ cup margarine
½ cup buttermilk

4 tablespoons cocoa
½ cup shortening
½ cup water
2 eggs, beaten
1 teaspoon vanilla

- Preheat oven to 400 degrees.

- Mix flour, sugar, cinnamon, and soda in large bowl; set aside.

- In saucepan, mix margarine, buttermilk, cocoa, shortening, and water. Heat to rolling boil. Add to dry ingredients and mix well. Add 2 beaten eggs and vanilla. Pour into greased 13x9x2-inch baking dish and bake 20 minutes.

Frosting:
½ cup margarine, melted
4 tablespoons cocoa
6 tablespoons milk

1 (16-ounce) box confectioners' sugar
1 teaspoon vanilla

- Combine ingredients and mix well.

Very rich. Stays moist for 7 days.

Mrs. Jack W. Hoelscher (Barbara)

German Chocolate Pound Cake

2 cups sugar
1 cup shortening
4 eggs
2 teaspoons vanilla
2 teaspoons butter flavoring
1 cup buttermilk

3 cups flour
½ teaspoon baking soda
1 teaspoon salt
1 (4-ounce) package German sweet chocolate, melted

- Preheat oven to 300 degrees.

- Cream sugar and shortening. Add eggs, flavorings, and buttermilk.

- Sift flour, soda, and salt. Blend into creamed ingredients and add melted chocolate. Pour into 10-inch greased and floured tube pan. Bake 1½ hours.

Mrs. Billy W. McCann (Betty)

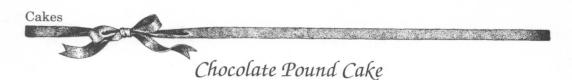

Chocolate Pound Cake

Cake:

½ cup margarine
½ cup Crisco
3 cups sugar
5 eggs
3 cups flour

½ teaspoon baking powder
¼ teaspoon salt
½ cup cocoa
1¼ cups milk
1 teaspoon vanilla

- Preheat oven to 325 degrees.

- Cream shortening and sugar; beat in eggs one at a time, blending well after each addition.

- Sift dry ingredients and add alternately with milk and vanilla.

- Pour into greased and floured 10-inch tube pan or bundt pan. Bake 1½ hours. Let cool 10 minutes before removing from pan.

Frosting:

1 (16-ounce) box confectioners' sugar
½ cup cocoa

½ cup margarine
4½ tablespoons hot coffee
1½ teaspoons vanilla

- Combine sugar and cocoa and cream with margarine. Beat in hot coffee and vanilla until spreading consistency.

Mrs. P. D. Miller, Jr. (Greene)

Mary T's Pound Cake

1 (16-ounce) box confectioners' sugar
2 cups butter
6 eggs

4 cups flour
½ cup orange juice
1 tablespoon vanilla

- Preheat oven to 300 degrees.

- Cream sugar and butter. Add eggs one at a time, beating well after each addition.

- Add flour alternately with orange juice and vanilla. Bake in greased and floured 10-inch bundt pan 1 hour and 15 to 20 minutes. Serves 12 to 16.

Mrs. David R. Libby (Donna)

Vanilla Wafer Cake

1 cup margarine, melted and cooled
2 cups sugar
6 eggs
½ cup milk

1 (7-ounce) package flaked coconut
1 cup chopped pecans
1 (16-ounce) box crushed vanilla
    wafers

- Preheat oven to 325 degrees.

- To margarine, add sugar, 6 eggs (one at a time) and milk. Blend in coconut and pecans, mixing well. Add vanilla wafer crumbs and pour into 10-inch greased and floured tube pan.

- Bake 1½ hours. Remove from oven, cool 10 minutes, then loosen edges of cake.

- Let set 20 to 25 minutes. Remove from pan, wrap in foil, and refrigerate.

Mrs. James F. Bigger, Jr. (Pat)

Coconut Pound Cake

Cake:
2 cups sugar
2 cups flour
½ teaspoon salt
1½ teaspoons baking powder
5 eggs

1 cup oil
½ cup milk
2 teaspoons coconut flavoring
1 (7-ounce) can angel flake coconut

- Preheat oven to 350 degrees.

- Mix all dry ingredients; add moist ingredients and coconut. Stir well by hand.

- Pour into greased and floured 10-inch bundt pan. Bake 55 minutes.

Glaze:
1 cup sugar
½ cup butter

1 cup milk
1 teaspoon coconut flavoring

- Combine ingredients in saucepan and simmer 2 minutes. Spoon over hot cake.

Mrs. Roy M. Smith (Katherine)

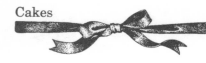

Coconut Cake

Cake:

2 cups sugar
1 cup shortening
5 eggs
2 cups self-rising flour, sifted

1 cup buttermilk
1½ teaspoons coconut flavoring
1 (3½-ounce) can flaked coconut

- Preheat oven to 350 degrees.

- Cream sugar and shortening. Add eggs, one at a time, beating well after each, until creamy smooth.

- Add flour and buttermilk alternately and beat 3 minutes. Add coconut flavoring and coconut. Beat well.

- Pour into greased and floured 10-inch tube pan. Bake approximately 55 minutes. Leave in pan and punch holes in top.

Topping:

½ cup water
1 cup sugar

1½ teaspoons coconut flavoring

- Combine ingredients and boil 1 minute. Pour over hot cake.

- Leave cake in pan until cool.

Mrs. H. Ray Manning (Rose Marie)

Ever So Easy Fruitcake

2½ cups unsifted flour
1 teaspoon baking soda
2 eggs, slightly beaten
1 (28-ounce) jar mincemeat

1 (14-ounce) can sweetened condensed milk
2 cups mixed candied fruit
1 cup coarsely chopped walnuts

- Preheat oven to 300 degrees.

- Generously grease and flour 10-inch tube pan.

- Sift flour and soda and set aside.

- Combine remaining ingredients in large bowl. Pour into prepared pan. Bake 1 hour and 50 minutes. Cool 15 minutes. Glaze as desired.

Mrs. Frank J. Hudson (Bettye)

Italian Cream Cake

Cake:

½ cup margarine
½ cup vegetable oil
2 cups sugar
5 egg yolks, beaten
2 cups flour
1 teaspoon baking soda

1 cup buttermilk
1 (3½-ounce) can flaked coconut
1 cup chopped English walnuts
1 teaspoon vanilla
5 egg whites, stiffly beaten

- Preheat oven to 350 degrees.

- Cream margarine and oil; add sugar and egg yolks.

- Combine flour and soda and add alternately with buttermilk. Add coconut, nuts, and vanilla. Fold in egg whites.

- Bake 25 minutes in 3 greased 9-inch baking pans.

Frosting:

1 (8-ounce) package cream cheese
½ cup margarine
1 (16-ounce) box confectioners'
    sugar

1 teaspoon vanilla
½ cup chopped English walnuts

- Cream together cream cheese and margarine. Mix in other ingredients. Ice cooled cake. Serves 15 to 20.

Mrs. Richard C. Harris (Beverly)

Lemon Nut Cake

2 cups margarine
2 cups sugar
6 eggs
4 cups flour

1 teaspoon baking powder
1 (15-ounce) box golden raisins
4 cups chopped pecans
2 ounces lemon extract

- Preheat oven to 275 degrees.

- Cream margarine and sugar. Beat in eggs one at a time. Add remaining ingredients.

- Bake 2 hours in two 9x5x3-inch loaf pans.

We prefer this to fruitcake at Christmas time.

Mrs. Justin D. Towner (Ginny)

Pineapple Upside Down Cake

1 cup brown sugar
1 (8-ounce) can sliced pineapple,
  drained and juice reserved
Maraschino cherries
Pecan halves
2 eggs, separated

4 tablespoons water
1 cup sugar
1 cup flour
2 teaspoons baking powder
⅛ teaspoon salt

- Preheat oven to 300 degrees.

- Put brown sugar and 4 tablespoons pineapple juice into 9-inch iron skillet and boil 2 minutes. Place pineapple slices, cherries, and pecan halves in pattern in syrup. Set aside to cool while making batter.

- Mix egg yolks and water. Add sugar, flour, baking powder, and salt.

- Beat egg whites until stiff and fold into batter. Pour over syrup and fruit. Bake 50 minutes. Turn onto plate. Serve with ice cream. Serves 6.

Mrs. Roy M. Smith (Katherine)

Rum Cake

Cake:
1 (18.25-ounce) box yellow cake mix
1 (3½-ounce) package instant
  vanilla pudding mix
½ cup light rum

½ cup water
½ cup vegetable oil
4 eggs

- Preheat oven to 350 degrees.

- Combine cake mix and pudding. Add rum, water, and oil. Add eggs one at a time, mixing thoroughly after each.

- Pour into greased 10-inch bundt pan. Bake 1 hour. Cool.

- Remove from pan and punch holes in top of cake.

Topping:
1 cup sugar
¼ cup water
½ cup butter

¼ cup light rum
Confectioners' sugar, optional

- Combine sugar, water, and butter. Boil 1 minute; cool and add rum. Pour over cake. Sprinkle with confectioners' sugar, if desired.

Best if made day before.

Mrs. Joe Hall Morris (Adair)

Fresh Strawberry Cake

Cake:

1 (18.25-ounce) box white cake mix
1 (3-ounce) box wild strawberry
 gelatin

½ cup vegetable oil
4 eggs
1 cup sliced fresh strawberries

- Preheat oven to 350 degrees.

- Combine all ingredients and beat two minutes in mixer. Pour in two 9-inch greased and floured cake pans and bake 25 to 30 minutes until cake tests done. Watch carefully.

Frosting:

½ cup margarine
1 (16-ounce) box confectioners'
 sugar

¼ cup sliced fresh strawberries

- Cream margarine and sugar well. Add strawberries and beat slightly until spreading consistency.

Miss Whitney Miller

Southern Dream Cake

1 (18.25-ounce) box Duncan Hines
 butter cake mix
1 (3¾-ounce) package instant
 vanilla pudding
1½ cups milk
1 (8-ounce) package cream cheese

1 (20-ounce) can crushed pineapple,
 drained
1 (21-ounce) can cherry pie filling
1 (8-ounce) carton Cool Whip
½ cup chopped pecans

- Prepare cake mix as package directs. Pour ⅔ mix into 13x9x2-inch greased baking dish. Bake according to package directions. Allow cake to cool after baking.

- Mix together pudding, milk, and cream cheese. Spread on top of cake. Next spread layer of pineapple, pie filling, and Cool Whip. Sprinkle nuts over top. Serves 15.

Use the remaining batter for a mini-cake or cupcakes.

Mrs. Dennis A. Sigman (Linda)

Almond Bark Goodies

1 (24-ounce) package white almond bark
2 tablespoons creamy peanut butter

1 cup Rice Krispies
1 cup miniature marshmallows
1 cup peanuts

- Melt almond bark in microwave or double boiler. Add peanut butter and mix well. Add remaining ingredients.

- Drop by teaspoon on waxed paper and let set. Makes 4 dozen.

Mrs. J. Howard McClain (Virginia)

Buckeyes

1 (16-ounce) box confectioners' sugar
½ cup butter (no substitute)
¼ bar paraffin

2 cups crunchy peanut butter
4 to 5 tablespoons milk
1 (6-ounce) package semi-sweet chocolate morsels

- Mix together with spoon or hands, sugar, peanut butter, butter and milk. Roll into small balls. These will be very stiff.

- Melt chocolate and paraffin together in top of double boiler. Spear each ball with toothpick and dip in chocolate, leaving some peanut butter showing at top.

- Place in refrigerator on waxed paper. If stored in tightly covered container, will keep indefinitely. Yields 7 dozen.

Mrs. John Winford (Sherrye)

Butterscotch Pralines

1 (4-ounce) package regular butterscotch pudding and pie mix
1 cup brown sugar, packed
½ cup sugar

½ cup evaporated milk
1 tablespoon butter
1 teaspoon vanilla
1 cup chopped pecans

- Mix first three ingredients. Add milk; stir well. Cook over medium heat until mixture comes to boil. Lower heat and continue cooking until candy reaches soft-ball stage when dropped in cold water.

- Remove from heat, add butter, vanilla, and pecans. Stir until candy begins to thicken. Drop from teaspoon onto greased cookie sheet.

This recipe makes a delicious caramel frosting for cakes or muffins.
Use same procedure as for pralines (leave out pecans).

Mrs. J. L. Eason (Mickey)

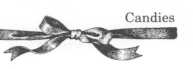

Chocolate Turtles

2 (16-ounce) packages caramels
4 tablespoons half-and-half
3 cups pecans
1 (6-ounce) package chocolate
** morsels**

2 chocolate Hershey bars
½ paraffin bar

- Melt caramels in cream. Add nuts and mix well. Drop by teaspoonfuls on foil covered 15x10x1-inch cookie sheet.

- Put in freezer while you melt chocolate morsels, Hershey bars, and paraffin on low heat.

- Dip "caramel bits" in melted chocolate mixture. Place candies back on pan and refrigerate overnight. Makes 4 dozen.

Mrs. James E. Sexton (Pat)

Fast Fudge

2 cups sugar
⅔ cup evaporated skim milk
12 large marshmallows
½ cup margarine or butter
⅛ teaspoon salt

1 (6-ounce) package semi-sweet
** chocolate morsels**
1 cup chopped nuts
1 teaspoon vanilla

- Combine sugar, milk, marshmallows, butter, and salt in a large saucepan. Cook over medium heat until it comes to boil, stirring constantly. Boil 5 minutes and remove from heat.

- Add chocolate, stirring until melted. Add nuts and vanilla.

- Spread evenly in buttered 8-inch square pan. Cut when cool. Yields 16 large squares.

Mrs. R. Malcolm Overbey (Mary Anne)

Vanilla loses flavor at high temperatures so remove pan from stove before adding vanilla to your recipe.

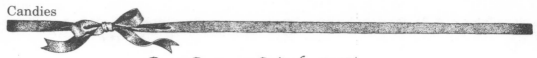

Best Peanut Brittle In Town

3 cups sugar
1 cup water
1 cup light corn syrup
⅛ teaspoon salt

¼ cup margarine
2 cups raw Spanish peanuts
2 tablespoons baking soda

- Combine all ingredients except peanuts and baking soda in heavy saucepan. Cook to 200 degrees.

- Add peanuts and cook to 300 degrees stirring constantly.

- Remove from heat. Add baking soda and stir quickly. Pour into two 15x10x1-inch jelly-roll pans. After candy cools, use knife handle to break into pieces.

Cookbook Committee

Peanut Butter Fingers

1 cup graham cracker crumbs
1 (16-ounce) box confectioners'
  sugar
1 (7-ounce) can flaked coconut
1 cup butter
½ cup peanut butter

½ teaspoon salt
1 teaspoon vanilla
1 cup chopped nuts
¼ block paraffin, melted
1 (6-ounce) package chocolate
  morsels

- Mix together all of the above ingredients except paraffin and chocolate. Roll in 2-inch fingers. Freeze. Take out of freezer and dip into melted paraffin and chocolate morsel mixture.

Mrs. James R. Smith (Peggy)

Chocolate Fruit Crunchies

3 tablespoons unsweetened cocoa
2 tablespoons butter or margarine
¼ cup light corn syrup
1 tablespoon orange juice

2 cups granola cereal
½ cup finely chopped dried apricots
½ cup raisins
⅔ cup crushed granola cereal

- Blend cocoa and butter. Stir in syrup and juice. Add 2 cups cereal and fruit.

- Blend with hands until mixed, and shape with cold moist hands into 1-inch balls.

- Roll in crushed cereal and store in airtight container. Makes 3 dozen.

Mrs. Ernest H. Sigman, Jr. (Doris)

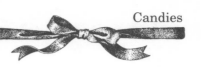

Orange Balls

1 (6-ounce) can frozen orange juice, thawed
1 (16-ounce) box confectioners' sugar
½ cup margarine, melted

1 (12-ounce) box vanilla wafers, crushed
½ cup chopped pecans
1 (7-ounce) package flaked coconut

- Combine first 5 ingredients and roll in small balls.

- Roll balls in coconut. Keeps well stored in tin in refrigerator.

Variation: Add 1 tablespoon lemon juice and ⅛ teaspoon salt with some grated orange or lemon peel for extra zip!

Mrs. Norman Towbin (Barbara)

Rocky Road

1 (12-ounce) package chocolate morsels
1 (14-ounce) can sweetened condensed milk

2 tablespoons margarine
1 (10½-ounce) package miniature marshmallows
1 (8-ounce) jar unsalted peanuts

- Melt chocolate morsels, condensed milk, and margarine. Combine marshmallows and peanuts. Blend all together.

- Spread mixture into 13x9x2-inch pan lined with waxed paper. Refrigerate several hours; cut into squares. Makes 48 small or 24 large squares.

Mrs. Sidney Friedman, Jr. (Ann)

Sweet Nothings

½ cup peanut butter
½ cup margarine
1 (6-ounce) package chocolate morsels

1 (12-ounce) box Rice Chex cereal
1 (16-ounce) box confectioners' sugar

- Melt first 3 ingredients in large pan on low heat. Remove from heat and stir in cereal until coated.

- Put sugar in grocery bag. Pour in coated cereal and shake, shake, shake! Yields 20 to 24 cups.

Mrs. Lee E. Wilson (Carol)

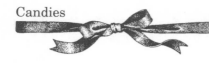

Skedaddles

1 (3-ounce) can chow mein noodles
1 cup miniature marshmallows
¾ cup sugar
½ cup evaporated milk

2 tablespoons butter
1 (6-ounce) package semi-sweet or
    mint flavored chocolate morsels

- Mix noodles and marshmallows in large bowl. Set aside.

- Combine sugar, evaporated milk, and butter in saucepan; bring to rolling boil over high heat, stirring constantly. Remove from heat and add chocolate morsels. Stir until melted. Let stand 15 minutes.

- Pour chocolate sauce over noodle mixture. Stir until well coated and drop by heaping teaspoonfuls onto waxed paper lined cookie sheets. Chill until set, about 1 hour. Remove from waxed paper. Makes about 2½ dozen.

Variations: Decrease evaporated milk to 6 tablespoons. Substitute 1 package butterscotch or milk chocolate morsels for the semi-sweet.

Mrs. John S. Buchignani, Sr. (Lutie)

Margaret's Granola

½ cup unsalted sunflower seeds
½ cup unsalted pumpkin seeds
½ cup sesame seeds
½ cup sliced almonds
½ cup cashew pieces
½ cup soy granola (TVP)

½ cup raw wheat germ
½ cup powdered milk
½ cup honey
½ cup safflower oil
2½ cups old fashioned oats

- Preheat oven to 300 degrees.

- Mix dry ingredients. Add honey and oil. Mix thoroughly.

- Bake in large roasting pan 40 to 45 minutes until golden brown, stirring every 10 minutes.

- Dry on brown paper. Store in air tight container. Will keep several weeks.

The Cookbook Committee

Date Crinkle Cookies

Filling:
1½ cups chopped dates
⅓ cup sugar

⅓ cup water

Dough:
1 cup shortening
1 cup brown sugar
1 cup sugar
1 teaspoon butter flavoring
2 eggs, beaten well
1 teaspoon vanilla

1½ cups flour
1 teaspoon salt
1 teaspoon baking soda
3 cups quick oatmeal
1 cup chopped pecans

- Cook filling ingredients in saucepan until thickened, stirring constantly.

- Cream shortening, sugars, and flavoring until fluffy; add eggs and vanilla and beat until mixed.

- Sift flour, salt, and soda and gradually add to other ingredients. Fold in oatmeal and pecans.

- Divide dough in half. On lightly oiled waxed paper, pat out dough until ¼-inch thick. Spread ½ of filling over dough. Roll in jelly roll fashion and wrap in waxed paper. Repeat process with other ½ of dough and filling.

- Chill in freezer 1 hour before slicing or freeze for several weeks.

- Preheat oven to 350 degrees.

- Slice thinly and bake on ungreased cookie sheets 8 to 10 minutes. Makes 8 dozen cookies.

Mrs. James R. Smith (Peggy)

*P*ack cookies for mailing by using popcorn to cushion plastic bags containing cookies.

Chocolate Chip Oatmeal Cookies

2 cups white sugar
2 cups brown sugar
2 cups margarine
4 eggs
1 teaspoon salt
2 teaspoons baking powder
1 teaspoon baking soda

2 teaspoons vanilla
4 cups flour
4 cups oatmeal, finely ground in blender
2 (12-ounce) packages chocolate morsels
3 cups chopped nuts

- Cream sugars and margarine; add eggs and beat well. Add salt, baking powder, soda, and vanilla; mix. Blend in flour, oatmeal, morsels, and nuts.

- Refrigerate at least 6 hours.

- Preheat oven to 400 degrees.

- Mold dough into golf size balls and place 2-inches apart on ungreased cookie sheet and press slightly. Bake 6 to 8 minutes. Freezes well. Yields 85.

Mrs. Phillip O. Dowdle (Evelyn)

Kourabiedes (Greek Cookies)

1 pound unsalted butter, softened
⅓ cup confectioners' sugar
1 egg yolk
3 drops anise, or 1 tablespoon bourbon

1 cup almonds, ground (optional)
2 to 2½ pounds flour
Whole cloves
Confectioners' sugar, sifted

- Preheat oven to 375 degrees.

- Beat butter well. Add ⅓ cup confectioners' sugar and egg yolk. Add flavoring and almonds.

- Add flour gradually. Knead by hand until dough is soft but not sticky.

- Pinch off small balls; roll into elongated shapes, then slightly flatten into crescent shape. Insert clove in center of each. Place on ungreased cookie sheet.

- Bake 30 minutes. Sprinkle heavily with sifted confectioners' sugar as soon as removed from oven. Makes 3 dozen.

Mrs. James G. Sousoulas (Sophie)

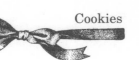

Pickwick Chocolate Chips

1 cup Crisco
1 cup firmly packed dark brown
  sugar
½ cup sugar
1 teaspoon vanilla
2 eggs

2¼ cups flour
1 teaspoon salt
1 teaspoon soda
1 cup chopped nuts
1 (12-ounce) package chocolate
  morsels

- Preheat oven to 375 degrees.

- Cream Crisco, sugars, and vanilla in mixer. Beat in eggs.

- Sift flour, salt, and soda. Gradually add to creamed mixture. Stir in nuts and morsels.

- Bake 8 to 10 minutes on greased cookie sheets. Makes 5 dozen.

Miss Traci Sherman

Lemon Crumb Cookies

2 cups flour, sifted
¼ teaspoon salt
1 teaspoon baking powder
1 cup butter
1⅓ cups light brown sugar
1⅓ cups old fashioned oats

1 (14-ounce) can sweetened
  condensed milk
½ cup lemon juice
1 teaspoon grated lemon rind
½ teaspoon salt

- Preheat oven to 350 degrees.

- Sift flour, ¼ teaspoon salt, and baking powder.

- Cream butter and sugar. Blend in flour mixture. Add oats and mix until crumbly. Spread ½ of this in 13x9x2-inch buttered baking pan and press firmly.

- Combine condensed milk, lemon juice, grated rind, and salt. Spread over crumb mixture and cover with remaining crumb mixture.

- Bake 25 minutes. Makes 36 squares.

Mrs. Walter Cooper Sandusky, Jr. (Lois)

*F*reeze citrus rinds for easier grating.

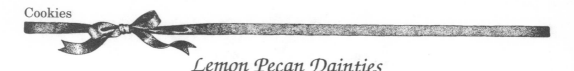

Lemon Pecan Dainties

½ cup shortening
1 cup sugar
1 egg, beaten
1 tablespoon lemon juice
1 tablespoon lemon rind

2 cups flour
1 teaspoon baking powder
⅛ teaspoon salt
1 cup chopped pecans

- Cream shortening; gradually add sugar, beating until light and fluffy.

- Add egg, lemon juice, and grated lemon rind; beat well.

- Combine flour, baking powder, and salt; add to creamed mixture, beating just until blended. Stir in pecans.

- Shape dough into long roll, 2 inches in diameter; wrap in waxed paper, and chill 2 to 3 hours or until firm.

- Preheat oven to 350 degrees.

- Unwrap roll and cut into ¼-inch slices; place on lightly greased cookie sheets. Bake 10 to 12 minutes. Makes about 3 dozen.

Mrs. Leon L. Bolton (Freddie Lou)

Nana's Jelly Centers

2¼ cups unsifted flour
½ cup butter
½ cup shortening
1 egg
¾ cup sugar

½ teaspoon vanilla extract
½ teaspoon almond extract
Seedless raspberry preserves
Confectioners' sugar

- Preheat oven to 350 degrees.

- Mix the first 7 ingredients. Shape into small balls and place on ungreased cookie sheet. If dough is too sticky to handle, add a little more flour.

- With forefinger, press down center of each cookie and fill with raspberry preserves.

- Bake approximately 15 minutes.

- Sift with confectioners' sugar while cookies are still hot. Yields 24.

Mrs. L. Carl Anderson (Maxine)

Oatmeal Crunchies

1 cup sifted flour
½ cup sugar
½ teaspoon baking powder
½ teaspoon baking soda
¼ teaspoon salt
½ cup brown sugar

½ cup shortening
1 egg
¼ teaspoon vanilla
¾ cup quick-cooking rolled oats
½ cup chopped black walnuts, or
   pecans

- Preheat oven to 375 degrees.

- Sift together flour, sugar, baking powder, soda, and salt. Add brown sugar, shortening, egg, and vanilla. Beat well and stir in rolled oats and nuts.

- Form dough into small balls and dip top in a little sugar.

- Place on ungreased cookie sheet. Bake 10 to 12 minutes. Makes 3½ dozen.

Mrs. Ernest Moore (Jane)

Praline Cookies

1⅔ cups flour
1½ teaspoons baking powder
½ teaspoon salt
½ cup butter

1½ cups brown sugar
1 egg
1 teaspoon vanilla
1 cup chopped pecans

- Preheat oven to 350 degrees.

- Sift flour, baking powder, and salt.

- Cream butter and brown sugar. Blend in egg, vanilla, and flour mixture. Stir in pecans. Drop onto ungreased cookie sheet. Bake 10 minutes.

Frosting:
1 cup brown sugar
½ cup evaporated milk

1 cup confectioners' sugar

- Combine brown sugar and evaporated milk in saucepan and boil 2 minutes. Blend in confectioners' sugar. Beat until smooth and drizzle on cookies. Yields 3 dozen.

Mrs. James F. Bennett, Jr. (Ann)

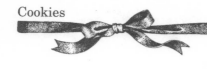

Raspberry Kisses

3 egg whites
⅛ teaspoon salt
3½ tablespoons raspberry flavored
  fruit gelatin powder

¾ cup sugar
1 tablespoon vinegar
1 cup chocolate morsels

- Preheat oven to 250 degrees.

- Beat egg whites with salt until foamy. Mix raspberry powder with sugar. Add gradually to foamy egg whites. Beat until mixture stands in peaks and sugar is dissolved. Mix in vinegar and fold in chocolate morsels. Drop by teaspoonfuls onto cookie sheets lined with brown paper.

- Bake 25 minutes. Turn off heat, but leave kisses in oven for another 20 minutes. Makes 7 dozen.

Mrs. J. Thomas Cobb (Ann)

Rocky Top Cookies

2 cups butter or margarine, melted
2 cups light brown sugar
2 cups sugar
4 eggs
2 teaspoons vanilla
4 cups flour
2 teaspoons baking soda

2 teaspoons baking powder
2 cups oats
2 cups crushed corn flakes
1 (6-ounce) package chocolate
  morsels
1 cup chopped pecans

- Preheat oven to 350 degrees.

- Blend butter and sugars. Stir in eggs and vanilla. Add flour, baking soda, and baking powder.

- Stir in oats, corn flakes, chocolate morsels, and pecans.

- Drop by heaping spoonfuls onto ungreased baking sheet.

- Bake 12 to 15 minutes. Makes 4 dozen big delicious cookies.

Mrs. James E. Sexton (Pat)

Egg whites will yield more volume if beaten at room temperature.

Sugar Cookies

1½ cups confectioners' sugar
1 cup margarine, softened
1 egg
1½ teaspoons vanilla

2½ cups flour
1 teaspoon baking soda
1 teaspoon cream of tartar

- Cream sugar, margarine, egg, and vanilla.

- Combine dry ingredients, add to creamed mixture and blend. Cover and refrigerate at least 3 hours.

- Preheat oven to 350 degrees.

- Place dough on lightly floured waxed paper. Cover with another sheet of waxed paper and roll to ¼-inch thickness. Cut and bake on ungreased cookie sheet 7 to 10 minutes. Yields 3 dozen.

Mrs. P. D. Miller, Jr. (Greene)
Mrs. David K. Rowe (Margaret)

Swiss Doubles

1 cup butter
1 cup sugar
2 egg yolks
1 teaspoon grated lemon rind
2 teaspoons freshly squeezed lemon
   juice

1 teaspoon vanilla
2 cups flour
Raspberry jam or apricot preserves
Confectioners' sugar, sifted

- Cream butter and sugar. Add egg yolks, lemon rind, lemon juice, and vanilla, blending well. Beat in flour. Chill dough.

- Preheat oven to 325 degrees.

- When ready to bake, remove small portion of dough at a time from refrigerator. Roll out to ¼-inch thickness on lightly floured board. Cut into desired shapes. Place on ungreased baking sheet. Bake about 15 minutes.

- When cookies are cool, put together (flat sides together) with raspberry jam or apricot preserves as filling to make sandwiches. Dust liberally with sifted confectioners' sugar.

- Makes 3 dozen. Freezes well.

Triple recipe for tea for 40 to 50.

Mrs. Robert K. Armstrong (Betty)

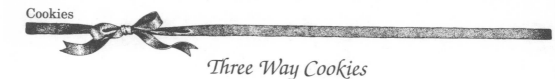

Three Way Cookies

1 cup shortening
½ cup sugar
½ cup brown sugar
2 eggs, separated
1 tablespoon cold water
1 teaspoon vanilla
2 cups flour

¼ teaspoon salt
1 teaspoon baking powder
½ teaspoon baking soda
1 (12-ounce) package chocolate
  morsels
½ cup brown sugar

- Preheat oven to 350 degrees.

- Cream shortening and sugars. Add egg yolks, water, and vanilla.

- Add flour, salt, baking powder, and soda and mix. Spread this mixture in a 13x9x2-inch pan. Sprinkle chocolate morsels over dough.

- Beat egg whites until stiff then gradually add ½ cup brown sugar and spread on top of chocolate morsels. Bake 30 minutes and cool. Cut into 18 squares.

Mrs. P. D. Miller, Jr. (Greene)

Lacy Cookies

1 cup margarine
1 cup sugar
1 cup brown sugar
2 eggs

1 teaspoon baking powder
1 teaspoon vanilla
2 cups oats
1 cup chopped pecans

- Preheat oven to 375 degrees.

- Combine all ingredients and mix.

- Drop by ½ teaspoonfuls on foil-lined cookie sheet.

- Bake 6 to 8 minutes. Lift foil to rack and cool. Gently peel foil from cookies. Makes 100 cookies.

Mrs. Roy M. Smith (Katherine)

For very thin rolled cookies, roll directly on bottom of a greased and floured cookie sheet. Cut the dough into shapes and remove surplus dough between them.

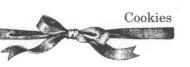

Blonde Brownies

¾ cup flour
3 teaspoons baking powder
⅛ teaspoon salt
1 (16-ounce) box light brown sugar
3 eggs, lightly beaten

⅔ cup oil
1 teaspoon vanilla
1 (6-ounce) package chocolate
  morsels
1 cup chopped pecans

- Preheat oven to 350 degrees.

- Mix flour, baking powder, salt, and sugar. Add remaining ingredients and pour into greased 15x10x1-inch jelly-roll pan. Bake 30 minutes. Yields 30.

Mrs. Jack Wohrman, Sr. (Jane)

Bumpy Brownies

2 ounces unsweetened chocolate
6 ounces semi-sweet chocolate
2 tablespoons butter
¼ cup flour
¼ teaspoon baking powder
⅛ teaspoon salt
2 eggs

¾ cup sugar
2 teaspoons instant dry coffee
½ teaspoon vanilla
6 ounces semi-sweet chocolate
  morsels
2¼ cups chopped pecans

- Preheat oven to 350 degrees.

- Melt unsweetened chocolate, semi-sweet chocolate, and butter.

- Sift flour, baking powder, and salt. Stir into melted chocolate mixture.

- Beat eggs, sugar, coffee, and vanilla together; add to above mixture.

- Stir chocolate morsels and pecans into batter by hand.

- Drop on foil lined cookie sheet. Bake 10 to 12 minutes. Be sure not to over bake. Makes 3 dozen.

Mrs. William O. Coley, Jr. (Fran)

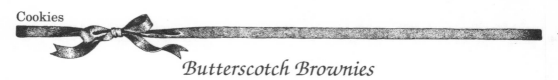

Butterscotch Brownies

Brownies:
4 tablespoons butter, melted
1 cup dark brown sugar
1 egg
½ teaspoon salt
¾ cup flour

1 teaspoon baking powder
½ teaspoon vanilla
¼ cup flaked coconut
½ cup chopped pecans

- Preheat oven to 350 degrees.

- Mix all ingredients and spread in buttered 8-inch square pan.

- Bake 25 minutes. Cool and spread with icing.

Caramel Icing:
½ cup butter
½ cup brown sugar
¼ cup half-and-half

1¾ to 2 cups confectioners' sugar
1 teaspoon maple or vanilla extract

- Melt butter until brown. Add brown sugar and cook, stirring until sugar is completely melted. Pour in half-and-half and stir. Cool.

- Add confectioners' sugar and extract. Beat until thick enough to spread.

Mrs. Bernard L. Rainey (Marjorie)
Mrs. James G. Avery (Karen)
Mrs. Leon L. Bolton (Freddie Lou)

Cup Cake Brownies

4 (1-ounce) squares semi-sweet
** chocolate**
1 cup butter
1 cup flour

1¾ cups sugar
4 eggs
2 teaspoons vanilla
2 cups chopped pecans

- Preheat oven to 325 degrees.

- Melt chocolate and butter together. Set aside.

- Mix flour and sugar. Add eggs, one at a time, stirring as little as possible.

- Add vanilla, chocolate mixture, and pecans, continuing to use a spoon to mix. Pour into paper baking cups in muffin pans.

- Bake 25 to 30 minutes. Do not over bake. Makes 24.

No mixer needed - just a spoon to mix.

Mrs. L. Carl Anderson (Maxine)

Fudge Brownie Bonbons

1 ounce square unsweetened
  chocolate
4 (1-ounce) squares semi-sweet
  chocolate
8 tablespoons butter
⅔ cup sugar
¼ teaspoon salt
2 tablespoons light corn syrup

½ teaspoon vanilla
¼ teaspoon almond extract
2 eggs
½ cup sifted flour
Garnish: whipped cream, blanched
  almond slices, candied cherry
  slices

- Preheat oven to 400 degrees.

- Line mini muffin tins (1½-inch diameter) with paper liners.

- Melt unsweetened and semi-sweet chocolate and 2 tablespoons butter over low heat; blend thoroughly.

- Beat remaining butter in medium bowl until fluffy. Gradually add sugar, salt, corn syrup, vanilla, and extract.

- Beat in eggs one at a time. Stir in melted chocolate mixture. Fold in flour.

- Spoon into muffin cups, filling ¾ full, and bake 10 to 12 minutes. Cool. Yields 3½ dozen.

- Garnish with whipped cream, blanched almond slices, and sliver of candied cherry.

Mrs. Mark E. Wiygul (Jan)

Boom Town Bliss Brownies

1 (18.25-ounce) box German
  chocolate cake mix
1 egg
½ cup margarine, softened
1 cup chopped pecans (optional)

1 (16-ounce) box confectioners'
  sugar, sifted with 2 tablespoons
  reserved
1 (8-ounce) package cream cheese
2 eggs

- Preheat oven to 350 degrees.

- Combine cake mix, 1 egg, margarine, and pecans; pat into greased and floured 13x9x2-inch baking pan.

- Combine confectioners' sugar, cream cheese, and 2 eggs and mix well. Spoon over cake mix layer. Sift reserved 2 tablespoons confectioners' sugar over top. Bake 40 to 50 minutes. Cool and cut into squares. Makes 15 to 20 squares.

Mrs. Leslie H. Binkley, Jr. (Nancy)

Mint Chocolate Brownies

Brownies:

½ cup butter or margarine
1 cup sugar
4 eggs
1 cup flour

1 (16-ounce) can chocolate syrup
1 teaspoon vanilla
4 tablespoons bourbon (optional)

- Preheat oven to 350 degrees.

- Cream butter and sugar; add eggs, flour, syrup, and vanilla and mix well. Pour into greased 13x9x2-inch baking pan.

- Bake 25 minutes. Pour bourbon on hot brownies. Cool completely.

Icing:

½ cup butter or margarine,
  softened

2 cups confectioners' sugar, sifted
2 tablespoons crème de menthe

- Combine ingredients, cream well, and spread on brownies. Refrigerate.

Glaze:

1 (6-ounce) package chocolate
  morsels

2 tablespoons butter

- Melt morsels and butter together. Spread on top of icing. Refrigerate. Remove from refrigerator about 45 minutes before cutting into squares. Yields 36 brownies.

Mrs. Percy A. Bennett, Jr. (Dot)

Melt chocolate in microwave on high for 1 to 1½ minutes.

The term "bloom" refers to white or gray spots or streaks that you see when sugar or fat particles separate from chocolate. It does not affect the flavor or use of the chocolate.

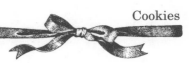

Geneva's Brownies

1 cup margarine
1 cup sugar
3 tablespoons cocoa
4 eggs

2 cups flour, sifted
1 cup chopped pecans
1 teaspoon vanilla
⅛ teaspoon salt

- Preheat oven to 350 degrees.

- Melt butter. Add remaining ingredients and beat by hand. Pour into greased 13x9x2-inch baking dish. Bake 25 minutes.

Frosting:
1 (16-ounce) box confectioners' sugar
5 tablespoons cocoa
6 tablespoons milk

4 tablespoons margarine, melted
1 teaspoon vanilla
⅛ teaspoon salt

- Beat ingredients together and spread on warm brownies.

Mrs. Walter Cooper Sandusky, III (Mona)

Presidential Brownies

1 cup butter
2 cups sugar
2 cups flour
⅔ cup cocoa

1 teaspoon vanilla
4 eggs
2 cups chopped pecans (optional)

- Preheat oven to 300 degrees.

- Put butter in 13x9x2-inch pan, melt in oven.

- Mix sugar, flour, and cocoa. Add melted butter, vanilla, and eggs. Mix well. Stir in pecans. Batter will be thick.

- Pour into buttered pan. Bake 30 minutes. Cool.

Icing:
1 (16-ounce) box confectioners' sugar
½ cup cocoa

½ cup butter, softened
1 teaspoon vanilla
5 to 6 tablespoons milk

- Combine all ingredients; mix well and frost brownies. Makes approximately 3 dozen.

Mrs. Malcolm Overbey (Mary Anne)

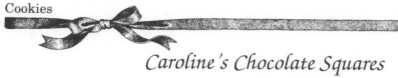

Caroline's Chocolate Squares

2 (1-ounce) squares unsweetened chocolate	2 eggs
½ cup butter or margarine	⅛ teaspoon salt
1 cup sugar	1 teaspoon vanilla
⅔ cup flour	¼ cup bourbon

- Preheat oven to 350 degrees.

- Melt together chocolate and margarine. Cool slightly; add sugar, flour, eggs, salt, and vanilla.

- Pour into greased 8-inch square baking pan. Bake 20 to 25 minutes. Remove from oven, and immediately pour bourbon over brownies. Cool.

Frosting:

2 cups confectioners' sugar	2 tablespoons rum
¼ cup margarine, softened	

- Combine frosting ingredients and spread over brownies.

Topping:

1 (6-ounce) package semi-sweet chocolate morsels	2 tablespoons margarine

- Melt chocolate morsels and margarine together and drizzle over brownies. Add few drops of water, if needed to thin. Makes 24 squares.

Mrs. Richard J. Reynolds (Anne)

Apricot Squares

1 cup margarine	2¼ cups flour, divided
¾ cup sugar	½ cup chopped nuts
1 egg yolk, beaten	1 (12-ounce) jar apricot preserves

- Preheat oven to 350 degrees.

- Cream margarine and sugar. Add egg yolk, 2 cups flour, and nuts. Set aside ½ cup dough and add ¼ cup flour.

- Spread remainder of dough on 15x10x1-inch jelly-roll pan. Bake 10 minutes. Cool. Spread jam on cooled crust. Sprinkle reserved dough on top. Bake at 325 degrees 20 to 30 minutes. Cut into squares while warm. Yields 3 dozen.

Mrs. Justin D. Towner (Ginny)

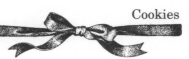

Applesauce Spice Squares

1½ cups whole wheat flour
1½ teaspoons baking soda
1½ teaspoons cinnamon
1 teaspoon cloves
½ teaspoon nutmeg
½ cup butter, softened

½ cup honey
2 eggs
2 teaspoons vanilla
1½ cups unsweetened applesauce
1 cup coarsely chopped walnuts
1 cup raisins

- Preheat oven to 350 degrees.

- Sift flour, soda, cinnamon, cloves, and nutmeg.

- Cream butter and honey. Add eggs, vanilla, and applesauce. At low speed, beat in flour mixture just until combined. Stir in walnuts and raisins. Pour into greased 13x9x2-inch baking pan.

- Bake 25 minutes or just until surface springs back when gently pressed with fingertips. Cool on wire rack. Cut into squares. Makes about 3 dozen.

Mrs. James L. Wiygul (Lou)

Flavoring extracts will be distributed evenly if they are added to the liquids.

Dusting walnuts with a little flour before mixing into batter prevents walnuts from sinking to the bottom.

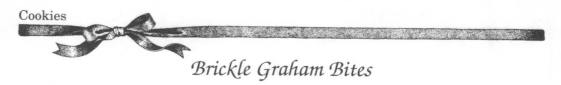

Brickle Graham Bites

14 to 16 whole graham crackers

• Line 13x9x2-inch baking pan with ½ the graham crackers.

Filling:

1 cup margarine, melted
1 cup sugar
1 egg, slightly beaten
¼ cup milk

½ cup graham cracker crumbs
½ cup Bits O' Brickle
½ cup chopped pecans

• Mix margarine, sugar, egg, and milk and bring to full boil, stirring constantly. Remove from heat and cool to room temperature.

• Add graham cracker crumbs, Bits O' Brickle, and pecans. Mix well. Spread over graham crackers in pan and top with remaining ½ of whole graham crackers.

Frosting:

¼ cup margarine
2 cups confectioners' sugar

Milk to moisten

• Combine ingredients and spread evenly over top of layers.

• Sprinkle with Bits O' Brickle for garnish. Cover and refrigerate overnight. Yields 64 small bars.

Mrs. Jerry A. Midyett (Beverly)

Dixie Bars

1 cup butter or margarine, softened
1 cup dark brown sugar
1 cup sugar
2 eggs
2 cups flour

½ teaspoon salt
1 teaspoon vanilla
1 cup pecans, chopped
Confectioners' sugar

• Preheat oven to 325 degrees.

• Cream butter and sugars. Add eggs and mix well. Add next 4 ingredients. Batter will be stiff. Spoon into buttered 13x9x2-inch baking pan.

• Bake 30 minutes. After removing from oven, sprinkle confectioners' sugar on top.

Mrs. Jerry A. Midyett (Beverly)

Nancy's Peanut Butter Cup Tarts

36 miniature Reese's peanut butter cups

1 (15-ounce) roll refrigerated peanut butter cookie dough

- Preheat oven to 350 degrees.

- Unwrap each piece of candy.

- Follow slicing instructions on cookie dough. Place each dough piece in greased miniature muffin cup pan.

- Bake 8 to 10 minutes or just until cookie puffs up and is barely done. Remove from oven and immediately push a candy cup into each cookie-filled muffin cup. The cookie will deflate and form a tart shell around peanut butter cup. The heat of the cookie will melt the chocolate topping.

- Let pan cool, refrigerate until shine leaves the chocolate, and gently lift out each tart with knife tip. Makes 36 cookies.

Mrs. Thad L. Morris (Barbara)

Butterscotch Cheesecake Bars

Crust:
1 (12-ounce) package butterscotch morsels
⅓ cup margarine or butter

2 cups graham cracker crumbs
1 cup chopped pecans

- In medium saucepan, melt morsels and margarine; stir in crumbs and pecans.

- Press ½ the mixture firmly in bottom of greased 13x9x2-inch baking pan.

Filling:
1 (8-ounce) package cream cheese, softened
1 (14-ounce) can sweetened condensed milk

1 teaspoon vanilla
1 egg

- Preheat oven to 350 degrees (325 degrees for glass dish).

- Beat cream cheese until fluffy; beat in condensed milk, vanilla, and egg. Pour into prepared crust and top with remaining crumb mixture.

- Bake 25 to 30 minutes or until toothpick inserted near center comes out clean.

- Cool to room temperature and chill before cutting into bars. Yields 15 to 20 bars.

Mrs. Jack C. Brooks (Betty Lou)

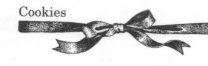

Date Nut Bars

1 cup flour
1 teaspoon salt
1 teaspoon baking powder
½ cup butter or margarine
1 cup sugar

2 eggs
1 teaspoon vanilla
1 (8-ounce) package chopped dates
1 cup chopped pecans
Confectioners' sugar

- Preheat oven to 350 degrees.

- Sift flour, salt, and baking powder.

- Cream butter, add sugar and eggs, one at a time; beat until fluffy.

- Blend in dry ingredients. Beat and add vanilla. Fold in dates and pecans.

- Spread into greased and floured 13x9x2-inch baking pan. Bake 25 to 30 minutes or until golden and firm. Cut while warm. When completely cooled, sprinkle with confectioners' sugar. Makes 15 to 20 bars.

Mrs. John Winford (Sherrye)

English Toffee Squares

1 cup butter
1 cup light brown sugar
1 egg yolk, slightly beaten
1 cup flour

⅛ teaspoon salt
1 teaspoon vanilla
6 (1.55-ounce) milk chocolate bars
1 cup chopped pecans

- Preheat oven to 350 degrees.

- Cream butter and sugar; add egg yolk, flour, salt, and vanilla; mix well. Spread into 13x9x2-inch baking pan.

- Bake 20 minutes. Remove and spread chocolate bars over top immediately. Sprinkle with chopped pecans.

- Chill. Cut into 4 dozen squares. Place in tin and refrigerate. Freezes well.

Mrs. John Mallett Barron (Doy)

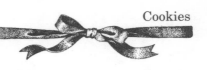

Toffee Bars

1 (16-ounce) box graham crackers
½ cup margarine
½ cup butter

½ cup sugar
¾ cup chopped pecans or 1 (2.25-ounce) package sliced almonds

- Preheat oven to 350 degrees.

- Cover a rimmed cookie sheet with aluminum foil. Break crackers into small bar pieces and lay on foil.

- Melt margarine, butter, and sugar and bring to boil. Boil 2 minutes. Pour over crackers. Sprinkle pecans or almonds on crackers.

- Bake 8 minutes. Cool slightly before removing from pan.

Mrs. J. D. Thomas (Donna)

Lemon Dessert Squares

2 cups flour
½ cup confectioners' sugar

1 cup margarine

- Preheat oven to 350 degrees.

- Sift flour and confectioners' sugar. Cream with margarine. Spread in bottom of 13x9x2-inch baking dish, patting down with fingers.

- Bake 20 minutes. Watch carefully so it will not get too brown.

Filling:
2 cups sugar
4 tablespoons flour
1 teaspoon baking powder
¼ teaspoon salt

4 eggs, beaten
5 tablespoons lemon juice
1 tablespoon lemon rind

- While crust is baking, combine filling ingredients and mix well.

- Pour filling into baked crust and bake 20 minutes. Cool, sprinkle with confectioners' sugar, and cut into squares. Serve plain or with whipped cream or ice cream. Yields 3 dozen.

These freeze well.

Mrs. Richard C. Harris (Beverly)
Mrs. Bruce H. McCullar (Jennifer)
Mrs. Justin D. Towner (Ginny)

Pecan Shortbread Squares

1 cup butter or margarine
1 cup sugar
2 cups flour
1 tablespoon cinnamon

⅛ teaspoon salt
1 egg white, beaten
1 cup chopped pecans

- Preheat oven to 350 degrees.

- Mix first 5 ingredients and pat to ¼-inch thickness on a greased 15x10x1-inch jelly-roll pan.

- Spread beaten egg white on top and sprinkle with chopped pecans. Bake 15 minutes and cut into squares while still hot. Yields 3 dozen.

Mrs. June Prichard Robinson

Caramel Tennessee Bars

1 (14-ounce) package light caramels
⅓ cup evaporated milk
1 (18.25-ounce) box German chocolate cake mix
¾ cup margarine, melted

⅓ cup evaporated milk
1 cup chopped nuts
1 (6-ounce) package chocolate morsels

- Preheat oven to 350 degrees.

- Combine caramels and ⅓ cup evaporated milk in double boiler; cook over low heat until caramels melt. Set aside.

- Stir dry cake mix, margarine, evaporated milk, and nuts in large mixing bowl. Press ½ of dough mixture into greased and floured 13x9x2-inch baking pan. Bake 6 minutes.

- Sprinkle chocolate morsels over crust. Spread caramel mixture over morsels; crumble remaining ½ of dough on top. Bake 15 to 18 minutes. Cool slightly and refrigerate 30 minutes before serving. Yields 24 to 36 bars.

Mrs. Jack W. Hoelscher (Barbara)
Mrs. Hampton H. Holcomb (Nancy)
Mrs. James B. Cochran (Linda)

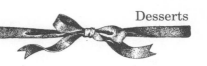

Baked Alaska

Day Before Serving:
6 (½-inch) thick slices pound cake, or 6 (½-inch) thick brownies, or 6 shortcake cups   1 quart ice cream, any flavor

- If using pound cake or brownies, cut with 2½-inch biscuit cutter. Place on foil lined cookie sheet and top each one with scoop of ice cream. Freeze.

Day of Serving:
½ cup egg whites   ½ teaspoon vanilla
½ cup sugar

- Beat egg whites until stiff; add sugar 1 tablespoon at a time, beating well after each addition. Add vanilla. Remove cakes topped with ice cream from freezer. Quickly and completely ice each one with beaten egg whites. Return to freezer at least 3 hours.

Ready to Serve:
1 cup chocolate sauce (see index)

- Preheat oven to 450 degrees.
- Remove Alaska from freezer and bake 1 to 2 minutes until slightly brown; top each one with warm chocolate sauce and serve immediately. Serves 6.

Easy and elegant dessert which can be made ahead of time.

Mrs. P. D. Miller, Jr. (Greene)

Banana Ice Cream

2 cups whipping cream   Juice of 3 lemons
2 cups half-and-half   2 cups orange juice
6 ripe bananas, mashed   2 bags crushed ice
1¾ cups sugar   1 (4-pound) box rock salt

- Combine whipping cream and half-and-half. Pour into ice cream freezer. Turn until chilled.
- Add bananas, sugar, and juices. Mix well. Freeze in ice cream maker according to directions using ice and salt. Serves 10 to 15.

Dr. Phillip Sherman, Jr.

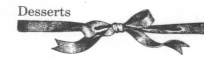

Apricot Freeze

1 cup vanilla wafer crumbs
  (22 wafers)
⅓ cup sliced almonds
3 tablespoons margarine, melted

1 teaspoon almond extract
1 quart vanilla ice cream, softened
12 ounces apricot preserves

- Combine crumbs, almonds, margarine, and extract. Reserve ¼ cup of this mixture for topping. Press remainder in bottom of 8 or 9-inch square baking dish.

- Quickly blend ice cream and preserves with mixer. Spread over crumb base. Sprinkle with remainder of crumb topping mixture.

- Cover and freeze at least 6 hours. Before serving, allow to set out about 15 minutes and soften slightly. Serves 8.

Mrs. Thomas C. Patterson (Margaret)

Frozen Chocolate Mousse

1⅔ cups graham cracker crumbs
⅓ cup margarine, melted
6 (1-ounce) squares semi-sweet
  chocolate, melted
3 eggs, separated, room
  temperature

1 teaspoon vanilla
½ cup chopped pecans
1½ cups whipping cream, whipped
  and divided
⅓ cup sugar

- Preheat oven to 350 degrees.

- Combine graham cracker crumbs and margarine. Press into bottom of 8 or 9-inch springform pan. Bake 10 minutes. Cool.

- Beat together chocolate, egg yolks, and vanilla. Stir in pecans. Reserve 1 cup whipped cream; blend remaining cream into chocolate mixture.

- Beat egg whites until foamy. Gradually beat in sugar until stiff. Fold into chocolate mixture and pour into prepared crust.

- Garnish with reserved whipped cream. Cover and freeze 6 hours or overnight. Serves 6 to 8.

Mrs. James R. Ross (Lucy)

Chocolate Peppermints

1 cup butter
2 cups confectioners' sugar
4 eggs
4 (1-ounce) squares unsweetened
   chocolate, melted

2 teaspoons vanilla
1 or 2 drops oil of peppermint
1 cup toasted chopped pecans

- Cream butter and sugar. Add eggs one at a time and beat well. Add melted chocolate, vanilla, and peppermint to taste.

- Sprinkle bottoms of approximately 20 paper muffin cups with pecans. Place cups in muffin tins and fill ¾ full with chocolate mixture. Freeze.

Variation: Place vanilla wafer in each muffin cup, fill with chocolate peppermint mixture and top with whipped topping, pecans, and cherries with stems.

Mrs. Winfield Dunn (Betty)
Mrs. Robert W. Hewitt (Betty)

Delta Ice Cream

8 eggs
2½ cups sugar
3 tablespoons cornstarch
1⅛ teaspoons salt

1 quart half-and-half
½ gallon milk
5 tablespoons vanilla

- Beat eggs in 8-quart sauce pot. Add sugar, cornstarch, and salt. Beat well. Slowly stir in half-and-half and milk.

- Cook over medium heat, stirring constantly, until mixture almost comes to boil, thickens slightly, and coats a silver spoon (about 180 degrees).

- Cool to room temperature, add vanilla and freeze in 5-quart freezer.

Dr. David R. Libby

Ribbon Layered Lemon Pie

¼ cup margarine or butter
⅓ cup lemon juice
¾ cup sugar
⅛ teaspoon salt

3 eggs, lightly beaten
1 quart vanilla ice cream
1 (9-inch) graham cracker crust

- In medium saucepan melt margarine and add lemon juice, sugar, and salt. Cook and stir until sugar dissolves.

- Pour hot lemon mixture slowly into eggs and return to saucepan. Cook and stir constantly until thickened. Chill.

- Put ½ of slightly softened ice cream in pie shell. Spread ½ of chilled lemon sauce over ice cream. Repeat layers. Freeze overnight. Garnish with strawberries. Serves 6 to 8.

Mrs. Richard C. Harris (Beverly)

Pineapple Sherbet

1 quart fresh lemonade, chilled
2 cups sugar
4 egg whites, beaten

1 (20-ounce) can crushed pineapple
1 quart milk

- Pour lemonade into 4-quart ice cream freezer and partially freeze.

- Combine sugar, egg whites, pineapple, and 2 cups milk. Add to partially frozen lemonade. If needed, add remaining milk to reach marked level in freezer. Freeze.

Mrs. Charles E. Harbison (Betty)

Tutti-Frutti Ice Cream

1 cup pecan halves
Juice of 3 lemons
Juice of 4 oranges
1 (15¼-ounce) can pineapple
   chunks, undrained

6 cups milk, or half-and-half
3 cups sugar
6 or 7 bananas, mashed

- Soak pecan halves in lemon juice, orange juice, and pineapple chunks. Add milk and sugar. Add mashed bananas. Freeze in 4-quart ice cream freezer. Serves 16.

Mrs. Stephen Weir (Dottie)

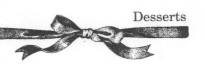

Peach Ice Cream

1 quart crushed very ripe peaches
1 cup sugar
Juice of 3 lemons

½ gallon milk
2 cups whipping cream
1 cup sugar

• Slice peaches into blender and crush to make 1 quart.

• Combine peaches, 1 cup sugar, and lemon juice. Set aside at least 15 minutes.

• Mix milk, cream, and 1 cup sugar in 6-quart freezer. Add peaches and freeze.

Mrs. Justin D. Towner (Ginny)

Vanilla Ice Cream

3 cups whipping cream
3 (14-ounce) cans sweetened
  condensed milk

3 (14-ounce) cans water
3 tablespoons vanilla

• Combine ingredients and freeze in ice cream freezer.

Mrs. Jack W. Hoelscher (Barbara)

Lemons heated in a microwave for 20 seconds release more juice when squeezed.

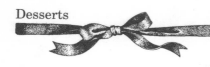

Cream Puffs

1 cup water
½ cup margarine
1 cup flour
¼ teaspoon salt

3 eggs
1 teaspoon vanilla
½ cup finely chopped pecans

- Preheat oven to 400 degrees.

- Heat water and margarine to rolling boil. Reduce heat. Stir in flour and salt until mixture forms ball (about 1 minute).

- Remove from heat. Add eggs, one at a time, then vanilla, and beat until mixture becomes shiny and smooth.

- Drop by teaspoonfuls on foil lined cookie sheet 1-inch apart. Bake 20 to 25 minutes until puffs are golden brown. Remove from oven and pierce side of each puff. Cool and frost with your favorite frosting. Sprinkle with pecans. Makes 4 dozen puffs. Freezes well.

Variation: Before frosting, puffs may be split and filled with your favorite custard. May omit vanilla, add one egg, split when cooked, and fill with chicken salad.

Mrs. Robert W. Hewitt (Betty)

Shortcake

2 cups flour
½ teaspoon salt
4 teaspoons baking powder
2 tablespoons sugar

⅓ cup margarine
1 egg
½ cup milk

- Preheat oven to 425 degrees.

- Mix all ingredients and roll out to 1-inch thickness. Cut with biscuit cutter. Arrange on cookie sheet and bake 8 to 10 minutes or until golden brown.

- Slice open and serve with fresh fruit and whipped cream. Makes 6.

Mrs. Frank J. Hudson (Bettye)

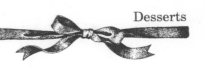

Apple Crisp

6 apples, pared, cored and sliced
1 cup sugar, divided
¼ teaspoon cloves
¼ teaspoon cinnamon
½ teaspoon nutmeg

2 tablespoons lemon juice
¾ cup flour, sifted
⅛ teaspoon salt
6 tablespoons butter
¼ cup chopped walnuts

- Preheat oven to 350 degrees.

- Place apples in bowl; add ½ cup sugar, spices, and lemon juice. Mix lightly; place in buttered 11x7x2-inch baking dish.

- Blend remaining sugar, flour, salt, butter, and walnuts until crumbly. Sprinkle over apple mixture. Bake 45 minutes or until apples are tender and crust is browned. Serve warm or cold. May be served with whipped cream if desired. Serves 6 to 8.

A good Thanksgiving fruit dessert.

Mrs. Bruce H. McCullar (Jennifer)

Apple Kugel

1 cup shortening
1½ cups sugar
1 teaspoon cinnamon
4 eggs
½ cup orange juice

1½ cups flour
1 teaspoon salt
6 apples, peeled, cored and grated
½ cup corn flake crumbs

- Preheat oven to 350 degrees.

- Cream shortening with sugar and cinnamon; add eggs and beat. Add orange juice, flour, and salt. Mix well. Fold in apples.

- Pour mixture into greased 9-inch square baking dish and sprinkle with corn flake crumbs. Bake 40 to 50 minutes.

Mrs. Danny Weiss (Saralyn)

No-Cook Banana Pudding

1 (6-ounce) package instant
  vanilla pudding
3½ cups milk
1 (14-ounce) can sweetened
  condensed milk

1 (8-ounce) carton frozen whipped
  non-dairy topping
Vanilla wafers
3 bananas

- Mix pudding mix and milk; add condensed milk. Fold in whipped topping.

- Layer vanilla wafers, bananas, and pudding. Repeat. Serves 6.

Mrs. Percy A. Bennett, Jr. (Dot)

Banana Split Dessert

2 cups graham cracker crumbs
1 cup margarine, divided
3 eggs, separated
2 cups confectioners' sugar
5 bananas
1 (16-ounce) can crushed pineapple,
  drained

1 (16-ounce) carton non-dairy
  topping
Nuts
Cherries

- Combine cracker crumbs and ½ cup melted margarine. Place in bottom of 13x9x2-inch baking dish.

- Combine 3 egg whites, beaten fairly stiff, confectioners' sugar, and ½ cup softened margarine. Pour over crumbs.

- Split 5 bananas lengthwise. Place over egg white layer; pour drained pineapple over bananas.

- Top with non-dairy topping and sprinkle with nuts and cherries. Refrigerate overnight.

Mrs. Richard C. Harris (Beverly)

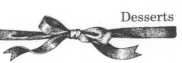

Bread Pudding with Lemon Sauce

¼ cup butter
4 eggs, beaten
1¾ cups sugar
1 teaspoon cinnamon
2 cups milk

5 slices white bread, or butter crust
   rolls, torn into pieces
½ cup white raisins
1½ teaspoons vanilla

- Preheat oven to 400 degrees.

- Melt butter in medium Pyrex bowl.

- In separate bowl, stir remaining ingredients together. Pour into 2-quart Pyrex bowl. Sprinkle top with more sugar and cinnamon.

- Put pudding in oven and immediately reduce heat to 350 degrees. Cook 55 minutes or until pudding is set.

Lemon Cream Sauce:
2 egg yolks
⅓ cup sugar
⅓ cup butter, melted

1 tablespoon grated lemon rind
3 tablespoons lemon juice
⅓ cup whipping cream, whipped

- Beat egg yolks until thick and lemon colored. Gradually add sugar. Add butter, lemon rind, and lemon juice.

- Fold in cream and chill in refrigerator.

- Spoon lemon sauce over pudding after it has been spooned into individual serving dishes. Serves 8.

Mrs. James F. Bennett, Jr. (Ann)

Mom's Boiled Custard

4 eggs
½ cup sugar
3 cups milk

¼ teaspoon salt
1 tablespoon vanilla

- Beat eggs with electric mixer. Add sugar gradually. Stir in milk, then salt. Cook in top of double boiler, stirring constantly, until custard coats silver spoon. Cover with waxed paper while cooling. When cool add vanilla. Makes 1 quart.

Dr. Graham H. Morris
Dr. Dwight A. Morris

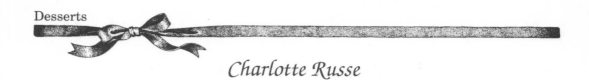

Charlotte Russe

2 envelopes unflavored gelatin
1⅓ cups milk
1 (32-ounce) carton whipping
  cream, whipped
4 eggs, separated

1½ cups sugar
2 teaspoons vanilla
Ladyfingers
1 (6-ounce) jar maraschino cherries

- Soak gelatin in milk; dissolve in top of double boiler.

- Whip cream until stiff and set aside in refrigerator.

- Beat egg yolks lightly with sugar. Beat egg whites until very stiff; add to yolks.

- Strain gelatin over egg mixture, stirring rapidly. Add vanilla; fold in whipped cream reserving enough for topping.

- Line bowl with ladyfingers; add charlotte and top with reserved whipped cream. Decorate with cherries and chill. Serves 8 to 10.

Mrs. Charles E. Harbison (Betty)

Flan

2 cups evaporated milk
1 cinnamon stick
1 lemon rind, grated
¼ teaspoon salt

6 egg yolks
3 egg whites
¾ cup sugar
1 teaspoon vanilla

- Preheat oven to 350 degrees.

- Bring milk, cinnamon stick, lemon rind, and salt to a boil. Remove from heat. Cool.

- Slightly beat yolks with egg whites, and add sugar and vanilla. Add milk mixture. Strain and pour into a caramel lined mold (directions stated below).

- Place mold in larger pan filled with approximately 1½-inches water.

- Cook in oven about 1 hour. Allow to cool before placing in refrigerator. Leave in refrigerator several hours before turning onto platter.

Caramel Lining:
½ to 1 cup sugar

- Cook sugar until it is caramelized and becomes like candy. Place in mold before custard ingredients.

Mrs. Fernando C. Heros (Gayle)

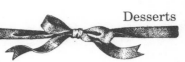

Brandied Caramel Flan

¾ **cup sugar**

- Preheat oven to 325 degrees.

- Place ¾ cup sugar in heavy skillet and cook over medium heat until sugar melts and forms a light brown syrup, stirring constantly. Immediately pour syrup into round 8¼-inch shallow baking dish. Holding dish with pot holders, rotate to cover bottom completely. Set aside.

Custard:
2 cups milk
2 cups half-and-half
6 eggs
½ cup sugar

½ teaspoon salt
2 teaspoons vanilla
2 tablespoons brandy (optional)
Boiling water

- In medium saucepan heat milk and half-and-half just until bubbles form around edge of pan. In large bowl beat eggs slightly; add sugar, salt, and vanilla. Gradually stir in hot milk mixture and brandy.

- Pour into prepared dish and set dish in shallow pan. Pour boiling water to ½-inch level around dish. Bake 35 to 40 minutes.

- Cool and refrigerate 4 hours or overnight. To serve, run small spatula around edge of dish. Invert on shallow serving dish. The caramel acts as a sauce. Serves 8.

Mrs. Joe Hall Morris (Adair)

Cranapple Crunch

2 cups fresh whole cranberries
3 cups chopped, unpeeled apples

1 cup sugar

- Combine ingredients. Put in buttered 3-quart casserole.

Topping:
1 cup quick oats, (not instant)
½ cup brown sugar

½ cup chopped pecans
⅓ cup margarine

- Preheat oven to 325 degrees.

- Mix oats, brown sugar, and pecans; place on top of cranberry mixture. Dot with margarine. Bake 40 minutes. Serves 10 to 12.

A delicious holiday favorite.

Mrs. J. Roy Bourgoyne (Helen Ruth)

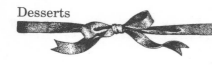

Fruit Pizza

1 roll refrigerated sugar slice-and-
bake cookies
1 (8-ounce) carton soft cream
cheese
⅓ cup sugar

½ teaspoon vanilla
Fruits of your choice
½ cup peach preserves
2 tablespoons water

- Preheat oven to 375 degrees.

- Slice cookie dough into fairly thin cookies. Completely cover pizza pan, overlapping cookies. Bake 10 to 12 minutes. Cool.

- Combine cream cheese and sugar and spread over cookie crust.

- Arrange assorted fruits in a decorative manner over the cream cheese mixture. Glaze with well mixed preserves and water. Serves 10 to 12.

Sliced bananas dipped in lemon juice, blueberries, grape halves, kiwi fruit, peaches, and strawberries are my suggestions for an appetizing presentation.

Mrs. Dwight A. Morris (Cathy)

Fresh Peach Soufflé

1 pound ripe peaches, pared and
cut into chunks
1 cup sugar, divided
1 envelope unflavored gelatin
⅛ teaspoon salt

Water
4 eggs, separated
¼ teaspoon grated lemon peel
2 teaspoons lemon juice
1 cup whipping cream, whipped

- Mash peach chunks coarsely. Stir in ¼ cup of sugar and let stand 1 hour, stirring occasionally.

- In top of double boiler combine gelatin, ¼ cup sugar, and salt.

- Drain syrup from peaches and add enough water to make ½ cup of liquid. Using a whisk, thoroughly blend egg yolks with peach liquid. Add this to gelatin mixture and cook over simmering water 4 to 6 minutes, stirring constantly. Remove from heat and add lemon peel and juice.

- Place top of double boiler in bowl of ice cubes, and stir mixture until it is slightly thicker than the consistency of egg whites. Stir in peaches. Add egg whites which have been beaten until stiff, but not dry, and sweetened with the remaining ½ cup of sugar. Fold into peach mixture. Fold in whipped cream last, then pour mixture into 2-quart soufflé dish and refrigerate 8 hours or overnight.

Mrs. James. R. Ross (Lucy)

Orange Fig Whip

1 cup whipping cream, whipped
1 cup broken fig newtons
1 (11-ounce) can mandarin orange
   sections, drained

½ cup chopped nuts

• Mix all ingredients lightly and chill. Serve in sherbet glasses. Serves 4 to 6.

Mrs. John Mallett Barron (Doy)

Four Step Pudding

½ cup margarine, melted
1 cup flour
1 cup finely chopped nuts
1 cup confectioners' sugar
1 (8-ounce) package cream cheese
1 (4-ounce) container frozen
   whipped non-dairy topping

2 (3¾-ounce) packages instant
   butterscotch pudding
3 cups milk
1 (8-ounce) container frozen
   whipped non-dairy topping
Nuts

• Preheat oven to 375 degrees.

• Mix melted margarine, flour, and nuts. Press into 13x9x2-inch baking dish. Bake 15 to 20 minutes.

• Mix confectioners' sugar, cream cheese, small whipped topping, and pour over crust.

• Make pudding using 3 cups milk instead of the 4 cups called for on package directions. Pour pudding over cream cheese mixture. Top with whipped topping and sprinkle with nuts.

Variation: Instead of butterscotch pudding, a mixture of 1 (3¾-ounce) package instant chocolate pudding and 1 (3¾-ounce) package instant vanilla pudding may be used.

Mrs. Buford F. Wallace (Jo Ruth)

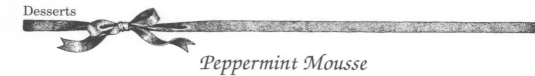

Peppermint Mousse

1½ tablespoons unflavored gelatin
2 cups milk
½ pound peppermint stick candy, crushed

½ teaspoon salt
1 cup whipping cream, whipped
Ground nuts, for garnish

- Soften gelatin in ¼ cup milk. Heat rest of milk in top of double boiler with candy.

- When candy melts, add gelatin, and salt. Dissolve well and cool quickly. When it begins to thicken, beat until light. Fold in whipped cream and chill. Spoon into parfait glasses. May be topped with ground nuts. Serves 6.

Mrs. L. C. Templeton (Virginia)

Raspberry Treat

3 egg whites
½ teaspoon cream of tartar
1 cup sugar
18 soda crackers
½ teaspoon salt

1 cup chopped nuts
1 tablespoon vanilla
1 (8-ounce) jar raspberry preserves
1 cup whipping cream, whipped
1 (6-ounce) package frozen coconut

- Preheat oven to 350 degrees.

- Beat egg whites until foamy. Add cream of tartar and beat until stiff. Fold in sugar, cracker crumbs, salt, nuts, and vanilla.

- Spread in buttered 13x9x2-inch pan and bake 30 minutes. Cool. Spread preserves over crust. Top with whipped cream and cover with coconut. Keep refrigerated. Serves 12 to 14.

A good make ahead dessert.

Mrs. Mark E. Wiygul (Jan)

Be sure beaters and bowl are well chilled when you whip cream.

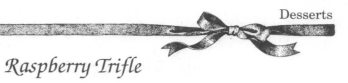

Raspberry Trifle

1 loaf pound cake
2 (12-ounce) jars raspberry
preserves

10 ounces raspberry liqueur

• Slice pound cake and spread raspberry preserves on each slice. Place slices back together and cut in cubes. Place cubes in covered air tight container and pour raspberry liqueur over cubes. Seal and let set overnight.

Custard:
2 tablespoons sugar
1 tablespoon cornstarch
2 large egg yolks

2¼ cups milk
½ teaspoon vanilla

• Place sugar and cornstarch in small, heavy saucepan (not aluminum); mix well.

• With small wire whisk, beat in egg yolks until you have a yellow paste. Gradually whisk in milk in a thin stream to prevent lumps.

• Place saucepan on medium heat, stirring with whisk until milk boils and thickens. Remove from heat and whisk in vanilla. Pour into storage container, cover with plastic wrap, and refrigerate until thoroughly chilled.

Next Day:
• Place layer of cake in trifle bowl. Pour custard over layer and repeat, ending with custard.

Garnish:
1 cup whipping cream, whipped
Frozen or fresh raspberries

Sliced almonds, toasted

• Top trifle layers with whipped cream, raspberries, and toasted almonds. Serves 8 to 10.

Mrs. James F. Bennett, Jr. (Ann)

For a curdled custard, slowly blend a beaten egg into the hot liquid.

Southern Sweet Chocolate Dessert

1 (4-ounce) package German sweet
  chocolate
¼ cup butter
1⅔ cups evaporated milk
1½ cups sugar
3 tablespoons cornstarch

⅛ teaspoon salt
2 eggs
1 teaspoon vanilla
1⅓ cups flaked coconut
½ cup chopped pecans

- Preheat oven to 375 degrees.

- Melt chocolate with butter in saucepan over low heat, stirring until blended.

- Remove from heat; gradually blend in evaporated milk.

- Mix sugar, cornstarch, and salt thoroughly.

- Beat in eggs and vanilla; gradually blend in chocolate mixture.

- Pour into 8x8x2-inch pan.

- Combine coconut and nuts. Sprinkle over filling.

- Bake about 55 minutes or until top puffs and cracks slightly. Cool at least 2 hours. Serve with whipped cream or ice cream. Serves 10 to 12.

Mrs. Gray Williams (Elizabeth)

Strawberry Compote

1 (13-ounce) angel food cake
1 (10-ounce) package frozen
  strawberries in juice
1 (6-ounce) package strawberry
  Jello

1 (6-ounce) package instant vanilla
  Jello pudding mix
3 large bananas, sliced
1 cup whipping cream, whipped

- Tear cake into small pieces. Place in bottom of large glass bowl.

- Mix strawberries and dry Jello together. Pour over cake.

- Make pudding according to package directions and spread over strawberry mixture. Add bananas and top with whipped cream. Serves 8 to 10.

Mrs. George H. Bouldien (Judy)

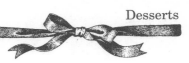

Strawberries Jamaica

1 (3-ounce) package cream cheese
1½ cups sour cream
½ cup firmly packed brown sugar

2 tablespoons Grand Marnier
liqueur
Fresh strawberries, sliced

- Cream first four ingredients in mixer and pour over strawberries.

*This is a light dessert served in individual dessert dishes
or cream may be served as a fruit dip.*

Mrs. James F. Bennett, Jr. (Ann)

Strawberry Lemon Dessert

12 to 18 ladyfingers, split
1 (14-ounce) can sweetened
condensed milk
1 tablespoon grated lemon rind

⅓ cup lemon juice
2 cups whipping cream, whipped
1 pint frozen or fresh strawberries

- Line bottom and sides of 2-quart springform pan with ladyfingers.

- Combine sweetened condensed milk, lemon rind, and lemon juice in large mixing
  bowl. Stir well. Fold in ⅔ of whipping cream and spoon into pan.

- Spread remaining whipped cream on top; cover and chill for 3 to 4 hours. Put
  strawberries on top before serving. Serves 8.

Mrs. James G. Avery (Karen)

Old Fashioned Strawberry Shortcake

2 cups self-rising flour
2 tablespoons sugar
½ cup butter
¾ cup milk

1 quart fresh strawberries,
sweetened to taste
1 cup whipping cream, whipped
and sweetened to taste

- Preheat oven to 425 degrees.

- Mix dry ingredients. Cut in butter and quickly stir in milk. Roll out on floured
  board to 9-inches in diameter. Place in two 9-inch round cake pans and bake 12 to
  15 minutes.

- Cool shortcake and then top one round with ½ of strawberries. Place second round
  on top and cover with remaining strawberries. Spread whipped cream over strawberries and garnish with a few extra berries. Serves 6 to 8.

Mrs. John Mallett Barron (Doy)

Strawberry Soufflé

2½ cups strawberry purée (1 quart
    fresh berries or 4 (10-ounce) boxes
    frozen)
2 envelopes unflavored gelatin
¼ cup water
⅔ cup sugar

4 egg yolks, well beaten
⅛ teaspoon salt
1 tablespoon lemon juice
4 egg whites
½ cup sugar
1 cup whipping cream, whipped

- Cut 3-inch band of waxed paper long enough to go around top of 1½-quart soufflé dish. Fasten to dish with tape.

- Purée strawberries in blender.

- Soften gelatin in water in top of double boiler. Add ⅔ cup sugar, egg yolks, salt, and 1 cup puréed berries, stirring well.

- Cook over boiling water about 5 minutes or until gelatin is dissolved. Remove from heat and cool slightly. Add lemon juice and remaining berries. Chill until consistency of unbeaten egg whites.

- Beat egg whites until frothy. Gradually add ½ cup sugar, beating until whites form peaks. Whip cream and fold into egg whites. Fold in chilled berry mixture and pour into prepared soufflé dish. Chill overnight.

- To serve, remove paper collar and garnish with additional strawberries and whipped cream. Serves 8 to 10.

Mrs. John Mallett Barron (Doy)

519

When separating an egg, if a bit of yolk gets into the white, remove with a piece of egg shell.

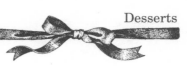

Easy Chocolate Sauce

¾ cup sugar
3 tablespoons cocoa
⅛ teaspoon salt
2 tablespoons water

1 (5-ounce) can evaporated milk
2 tablespoons butter
1 tablespoon vanilla

- In saucepan combine sugar, cocoa, and salt. Blend in water and stir until cocoa is dissolved.

- Add milk. Bring to boil. Cook 3 to 4 minutes. Remove from heat; stir in vanilla and butter. Makes 1½ to 2 cups.

Mrs. Phillip Sherman, Jr. (Sandy)

Gourmet Chocolate Sauce

¾ cup sugar
½ cup whipping cream
1½ tablespoons butter
2 (1-ounce) squares unsweetened
   chocolate

1 tablespoon brandy
¼ teaspoon vanilla

- Combine sugar, whipping cream, butter, and chocolate in saucepan. Cook over low heat until well blended. Increase heat to moderate and simmer 5 minutes undisturbed.

- Remove from heat and stir in brandy and vanilla. Serve warm. Makes 1 cup.

Mrs. David R. Libby (Donna)

Raspberry Sauce

1 (10-ounce) package frozen
   raspberries, thawed

1 tablespoon cornstarch
2 tablespoon cream sherry

- Drain raspberries, reserving juice. Put raspberries through food mill; discard seeds. Set berry pulp aside.

- Combine juice, cornstarch, and sherry in small saucepan; mix well. Cook over low heat, stirring constantly, until smooth and slightly thickened. Stir in raspberries. Cool. Yields 1 cup.

Serve over ice cream, custard or cake.

Mrs. James L. Wiygul (Lou)

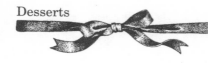

Caramel Icing

2½ cups sugar, divided
¾ cup half-and-half

2 tablespoons butter
1 teaspoon vanilla

- Put 2 cups sugar and half-and-half in saucepan and heat to boiling. At same time, caramelize ½ cup sugar in heavy saucepan. Add caramelized sugar to hot cream and sugar mixture, stirring constantly, until mixture forms firm ball when dropped in cup of cold water.

- Remove from heat; add butter and vanilla. Allow to cool. Beat until thick and ice cake. Will ice a 2 layer cake.

Mrs. Frank J. Hudson (Bettye)

Easy Milk Chocolate Frosting

3 tablespoon butter or margarine
2 tablespoons cocoa
1½ cups confectioners' sugar

2 tablespoons milk
1 teaspoon vanilla

- Melt butter or margarine in medium saucepan. Stir in cocoa until dissolved.

- Add confectioners' sugar, milk, and vanilla. Stir until smooth. Add more milk if necessary to make a soft spreading consistency. Makes enough frosting for 13x9x2-inch pan of brownies. Double recipe for frosting 2-layer cake.

Mrs. Charles B. Lansden (Ann)

Old Fashion Cocoa Frosting

**1 (16-ounce) box confectioners'
  sugar**
4 tablespoons cocoa

6 tablespoons butter, melted
5 to 6 tablespoons hot coffee

- Sift sugar and cocoa. Stir in butter and coffee until well blended. Do not beat. Will frost two 9-inch layers or 13x9x2-inch pan brownies.

Mrs. Charles E. Harbison (Betty)

Index

A

ACCOMPANIMENTS
Cornbread Dressing 228
Cranberry Chutney 38
Fresh Cranberry Sauce 226
Oyster Casserole 228
Pear Chutney 229
Pickled Okra 230
Pickled Pears 229
All-Bran Refrigerator Rolls 131
Almond Bark Goodies 260
Ambrosia Congealed Salad 96
Angel Biscuits 118
Angel Chocolate Pie 236
Ann's Cranberry Salad 89
Ann's Dill Bread 134
Antipasto 35
Anybody's Rolls 132

APPETIZERS

Cold
Antipasto 35
Avocado Mousse 36
Cheddar Cheese Ball 42
Cheddar Cheese Spread 41
Cheese Ring with Chutney 45
Cheese Wafers 43
Crab Pâté 52
Cucumber Cream Cheese Spread 37
Cucumber Mousse 37
Date and Cheese Rolls 39
Dill Dip 61
Dolmathakia (Stuffed
    Grapevine Leaves) 50
Easy Shrimp Dip 63
Elegant Pâté 45
Fancy Chicken Spread 46
Fresh Vegetable Mousse 59
Fresh Vegetable Squares 58
Fruit Dip 63
Green Bean Finger Sandwiches 55
Holiday Salmon Dip 63
Horseradish Mold 40
Layered Taco Dip 65
Mexican Tuna Dip 65
Mother's Cheese Wafers 44
My Caviar Cheese Ball 42
Party Pecans 59
Pickled Shrimp 54
Pimento Cheese Ball 42
Pineapple Cheese Ball 43

Plantation Cheese Ball 43
Seasoned Oyster Crackers 59
Sesame Cheese Straws 44
Shrimp Tomato Mold 51
Snow Peas with Boursin 54
Southern Crab Dip 51
Tea Sandwiches 56
Tuna Roll 65

Hot
Artichoke Dip 60
Asparagus Sandwiches 55
Baked Artichoke Hors d'Oeuvres 35
Baked Brie with
    Cranberry Chutney 38
Baked Chicken Nuggets 46
Barbeque Bologna 36
Broccoli Dip 60
Cheese Bacon Triangles 41
Chicago Artichokes 38
Cocktail Meatballs 47
Crab Rolls 52
Crabmeat Mornay 53
Croustades 39
Dip for a Crowd 61
Grilled Dove Breasts 39
Hot Bean Dip 61
Hot Crab Dip 62
Hot Tennessee Dip 64
Mini Reuben Sandwiches 56
Mushroom Turnovers 48
Nina's Clam Dip 62
Oysters Rockefeller 53
Quiche Individual 57
Sausage Stuffed Mushrooms 49
Sausage Swirls 50
Sesame Chicken Strips 47
Spinach Appetizers 58
Stuffed Mushrooms 49
Sweet and Sour Meatballs 48
Swiss Bacon Lorraine 57
Tiropetakia (Cheese Puffs) 40
Tomato Soup Dip 64

Sauces
Sweet and Sour Sauce 66
Tangy Dipping Sauce 66

APPLES
Apple Crisp 291
Apple Kugel 291
Apple Pie 233
Apple Strudel 117

Index

Apple-Butterscotch Sheetcake 245
Applesauce Spice Squares 279
Cranapple Crunch 295
Fresh Apple Cake 245
Harvest Apple Cake 246
Squash and Apple Bake 221
Stuffed Cornish Hens
   with Apple Dressing 187

APRICOTS
Apricot Bread 125
Apricot Freeze 286
Apricot Squares 278
Apricot Stuffed Pork 159
Baked Apricots 225
Swiss Doubles 271

ARTICHOKES
Artichoke Dip 60
Artichoke Lettuce Salad 90
Artichoke-Rice Salad 102
Baked Artichoke Hors d'Oeuvres 35
Chicago Artichokes 38
Shrimp, Mushroom and
   Artichoke Casserole 174

ASPARAGUS
Asparagus Casserole 205
Asparagus Sandwiches 55
Asparagus Soufflé 205
Asparagus Soup 75
Congealed Asparagus Salad 97
Aunt Dot's Lemon Carrots 209

AVOCADOS
Avocado Mandarin Green Salad 92
Avocado Mousse 36
Guacamole Salad Bowl 91

B

Bachelor's Dream Donuts 118
Bacon Quiche 202
Baked Alaska 285
Baked Apricots 225
Baked Artichoke Hors d'Oeuvres 35
Baked Bananas 225
Baked Beans Supreme 207
Baked Brie with Cranberry Chutney 38
Baked Brisket 147
Baked Chicken Nuggets 46
Baked Herb Tomatoes 223
Baked Orange Glazed Carrots 210
Baked Salmon Steaks 169

BANANAS
Baked Bananas 225
Banana Bread 126
Banana Cream Pie 234
Banana Ice Cream 285

Banana Split Dessert 292
Blackberry Jam Banana Bread 126
Fruit Salad with Banana Cream 88
No-Cook Banana Pudding 292
Barbecued Baked Beans 208
Barbeque Bologna 36

BAR COOKIES AND SQUARES
  (See Cookies)

BEANS
Baked Beans Supreme 207
Barbecued Baked Beans 208
French Market Soup 79
Hot Bean Dip 61
Bean Bundles 206

BEEF
Baked Brisket 147
Barbeque Bologna 36
Beef Stew with Beer and Walnuts 152
Chili Relleno Bake 158
Cocktail Meatballs 47
Company Eye of the Round 148
Company Meatloaf 153
Easy Five-Hour Beef Stew 151
Enchilada Casserole 152
Eye of Round Roast 149
George Washington Stuffed Roast 150
Gourmet Beef Tenderloin 148
Hot Tennessee Dip 64
Lasagna Casserole 156
Manicotti 155
Marinated Eye of Round Roast 149
Mary Ann Ward's Barbecued
   Brisket 147
Mini Reuben Sandwiches 56
Moussaka 154
Oven Swiss Steak 151
Quick Pepper Steak 149
South of the Border Salad 94
Stuffed Pasta Shells 157
Sweet and Sour Meatballs 48
Taco Casserole 153
Taco Salad 95
Tamale Casserole 157
Beets, Spicy 208
Best Coffee Can Dill Bread 135
Best Ever Chocolate Cake 251
Best Peanut Brittle In Town 262
Betty's Spiced Peaches 229

BEVERAGES
Blue Tail Fly 69
Mulled Wine 74

Punch
Champagne Punch 69
Coffee Punch 69

French 75 70
Fruit Punch... 70
Holiday Punch 70
Hot Rum Punch 72
May Bowl Punch 71
New Orleans Milk Punch 71
Percolator Punch 72
Pineapple Cranberry Punch 72
Sangría 73
Strawberry Punch 73
Uncle Henry's Milk Punch 71

Tea
    Lite Sun Tea 73
    Mint Tea 74
    Tennis Tea 74
Billy's Rye Bread 141
Black Russian Cake 246
Blackberry Jam Banana Bread 126
Blender Béarnaise Sauce 192
Blonde Brownies 273
Blue Tail Fly 69
Blueberry Lemon Tea Cake 127
Bonnie's Vegetable Soup 83
Boom Town Bliss Brownies 275
Boston Brown Bread 128
Bourbon Nut Bread 128
Brandied Caramel Flan 295

BREADS (See Cornbread and Muffins)

Fruit
    Apple Strudel 117
    Apricot Bread 125
    Banana Bread 126
    Blackberry Jam Banana Bread 126
    Blueberry Lemon Tea Cake 127
    Date Nut Loaf 127
    Lemon Nut Bread 131
    Plum Muffins 125

Miscellaneous
    Bachelor's Dream Donuts 118
    Boston Brown Bread 128
    Bourbon Nut Bread 128
    Buttermilk Biscuits 119
    Easy Monkey Bread 123
    Libby's French Pastry Log 130
    Spoon Bread 122

Spreads
    Fruity Cream Cheese Spread 144
    Strawberry Butter 144

Yeast
    All-Bran Refrigerator Rolls 131
    Angel Biscuits 118
    Ann's Dill Bread 134
    Anybody's Rolls 132

Best Coffee Can Dill Bread 135
Billy's Rye Bread 141
Bread Bountiful 137
Bread for Beginners 136
Grape Cluster 141
Harvest Sheaf 140
Jeanne Craddock's Rolls 132
Kate's Cream Cheese Braids 129
Khashapuri 142
Pocketbook Rolls 133
Sally Lunn Bread 134
Sour Dough Bread 138
Steamed Buns 143
Stuffed Bread 144
Whole Wheat Bread 139
Bread Pudding/Lemon Sauce 293
Brickle Graham Bites 280

BROCCOLI
    Broccoli Dip 60
    Broccoli Mold 108
    Broccoli Oriental Salad 104
    Creamy Broccoli Salad 104
    Fresh Broccoli-Cauliflower Salad 103
    Iced Broccoli Soup 75
    Joann's Broccoli Muffins 123
    Scalloped Broccoli Casserole 209
    Swiss Broccoli Soup 75

BRUNCH
    Angel Biscuits 118
    Apple Strudel 117
    Apricot Bread 125
    Bachelor's Dream Donuts 118
    Bacon Quiche 202
    Baked Apricots 225
    Baked Bananas 225
    Banana Bread 126
    Betty's Spiced Peaches 229
    Blackberry Jam Banana Bread 126
    Blueberry Lemon Tea Cake 127
    Boston Brown Bread 128
    Bourbon Nut Bread 128
    Buttermilk Biscuits 119
    Cheese Soufflé 199
    Date Nut Loaf 127
    Deviled Eggs and Ham 198
    Deviled Eggs with Mushrooms 197
    Dieter's Spinach Quiche 202
    Eggs Whitney 196
    Favorite Brunch Casserole 197
    Garlic Cheese Grits 196
    Hash Brown Potato Casserole 199
    Holiday Breakfast Casserole 196
    Honey Baked Fruit 226
    Hot Fruit Compote 227

Hot Gingered Fruit 227
Jo Ann's Broccoli Muffins 123
Kate's Cream Cheese Braids 129
Lemon Nut Bread 131
Libby's French Pastry Log 130
Oatmeal Muffins 124
Party Muffins 124
Piña Colada Muffins 124
Pineapple Cheese Casserole 230
Plantation Coffee Cake 119
Plum Muffins 125
Poppyseed Coffee Cake 120
Sausage Cheese Crescent
    Squares 200
Sausage Grits Casserole 200
Sausage Rice Casserole 201
Sausage Surprise 201
Buckeyes 260
Buffet Mixed Vegetables 213
Bumpy Brownies 273
Butter Roast Chicken 176
Buttermilk Biscuits 119
Butterscotch Brownies 274
Butterscotch Cheesecake Bars 281
Butterscotch Pralines 260

C

CABBAGE
Corn Slaw 105
Hot Slaw 106
Sauerkraut Salad 107
Savory Summer Salad 107
Sweet and Sour Slaw 106
Virginia's Corn Slaw 106
Caesar Salad 91

CAKES
Apple-Butterscotch Sheetcake 245
Best Ever Chocolate Cake 251
Black Russian Cake 246
Carrot Cake 247
Chocolate Chip Date Cake 252
Chocolate Fudge Oreo
    Sundae Cake 251
Chocolate Marshmallow Cake 250
Chocolate Pound Cake 254
Chocolate Sheetcake 253
Cocoa Cheesecake 248
Coconut Cake 256
Coconut Pound Cake 255
Ever So Easy Fruitcake 256
Favorite Cheesecake 249
Fresh Apple Cake 245
Fresh Strawberry Cake 259
German Chocolate Pound Cake 253

Harvest Apple Cake 246
Italian Cream Cake 257
Lemon Nut Cake 257
Mary T's Pound Cake 254
Mini Cheesecakes 250
Old Fashioned Strawberry
    Shortcake 301
Pineapple Upside Down Cake 258
Plantation Coffee Cake 119
Poppyseed Coffee Cake 120
Richglen's Cheddar Cheesecake
    with Strawberries 247
Rum Cake 258
Southern Dream Cake 259
Vanilla Wafer Cake 255
Calico Vegetable Salad 105

CANDY
Almond Bark Goodies 260
Best Peanut Brittle In Town 262
Buckeyes 260
Butterscotch Pralines 260
Chocolate Fruit Crunchies 262
Chocolate Turtles 261
Fast Fudge 261
Margaret's Granola 264
Orange Balls 263
Peanut Butter Fingers 262
Rocky Road 263
Skedaddles 264
Sweet Nothings 263
Caramel Icing 304
Caramel Tennessee Bars 284
Caroline's Chocolate Squares 278

CARROTS
Aunt Dot's Lemon Carrots 209
Baked Orange Glazed Carrots 210
Carrot Cake 247
Carrot Pudding 210
Champagne Punch 69
Charlemagne Salad 90
Charlotte Russe 294
Cheddar Cheese Ball 42
Cheddar Cheese Spread 41

CHEESE
Baked Brie with Cranberry
    Chutney 38
Butterscotch Cheesecake Bars 281
Cheddar Cheese Ball 42
Cheddar Cheese Spread 41
Cheese Bacon Triangles 41
Cheese Ring with Chutney 45
Cheese Soufflé 199
Cheese Soup 76
Cheese Wafers 43

Cheesy Stuffed Potatoes 215
Cocoa Cheesecake 248
Cucumber Cream Cheese Spread 37
Date and Cheese Rolls 39
Dip for a Crowd 61
Favorite Cheesecake 249
Fruity Cream Cheese Spread 144
Garlic Cheese Grits 196
Kate's Cream Cheese Braids 129
Mini Cheesecakes 250
Mother's Cheese Wafers 44
My Caviar Cheese Ball 42
Pimento Cheese Ball 42
Pineapple Cheese Ball 43
Pineapple Cheese Casserole 230
Pineapple Cream Cheese Pie 242
Plantation Cheese Ball 43
Richglen's Cheddar Cheesecake
    with Strawberries 247
Sausage Cheese Crescent Squares 200
Sesame Cheese Straws 44
Snow Peas with Boursin 54
Swiss Bacon Lorraine 57
Tiropetakia (Cheese Puffs) 40
Chicago Artichokes 38

CHICKEN
Baked Chicken Nuggets 46
Butter Roast Chicken 176
Chicken a la Crème 176
Chicken and Rice Delight 177
Chicken Breasts Supreme 177
Chicken Cranberry Layer Salad 96
Chicken Crescents 179
Chicken Enchilada Casserole 178
Chicken Florentine 180
Chicken Indienne 181
Chicken Marengo 180
Chicken Marsala 178
Company Chicken Divan 182
Cornish Hen with
    Raspberry-Sesame Sauce 188
Dip for a Crowd 61
Easy Chicken and Rice 181
Elegant Pâté 45
Fancy Chicken Spread 46
Hawaiian Chicken Salad 87
Hot Chicken Salad I 182
Hot Chicken Salad II 183
Karen's Chicken Soufflé 183
Louisiana Chicken Spaghetti
    for a Crowd 184
Mallett's Brunswick Stew 80
Nanny's Chicken Pot Pie 185
O'Farrell's Chicken Stew 184

Parmesan Chicken 185
Quick and Easy Chicken Delight 187
Rainbow Pasta Salad 111
Sesame Chicken Strips 47
Southern Fried Chicken 186
Stuffed Cornish Hens with
    Apple Dressing 187
Sweet and Sour Chicken 186
Chili Relleno Bake 158

CHOCOLATE
Angel Chocolate Pie 236
Best Ever Chocolate Cake 251
Black Russian Cake 246
Blonde Brownies 273
Boom Town Bliss Brownies 275
Buckeyes 260
Bumpy Brownies 273
Caramel Tennessee Bars 284
Caroline's Chocolate Squares 278
Chocolate Chess Pie 237
Chocolate Chip Date Cake 252
Chocolate Chip Oatmeal Cookies 266
Chocolate Fruit Crunchies 262
Chocolate Fudge Oreo
    Sundae Cake 251
Chocolate Fudge Pie 235
Chocolate Marshmallow Cake 250
Chocolate Peppermints 287
Chocolate Pound Cake 254
Chocolate Sheetcake 253
Chocolate Turtles 261
Cocoa Cheesecake 248
Cocoa Cream Pie 235
Cup Cake Brownies 274
Delta Chocolate Pie 238
Easy Chocolate Sauce 303
Easy Milk Chocolate Frosting 304
English Toffee Squares 282
Fast Fudge 261
French Silk Chocolate Pie 237
Frozen Chocolate Mousse 286
Fudge Brownie Bonbons 275
Fudge Pie 236
Geneva's Brownies 277
German Chocolate Pound Cake 253
Gourmet Chocolate Sauce 303
Mint Chocolate Brownies 276
Nancy's Peanut Butter Cup Tarts 281
Old Fashion Cocoa Frosting 304
Pickwick Chocolate Chips 267
Presidential Brownies 277
Rocky Road 263
Rocky Top Cookies 270
Southern Sweet Chocolate Dessert 300

Sweet Nothings 263
Three Way Cookies 272
"Watch Your Weight"
  Chocolate Cream Pie 238
Cindy's Marinara Sauce 194
Clam Dip, Nina's 62
Clear Tomato Soup 83
Cocktail Meatballs 47
Cocoa Cheesecake 248
Cocoa Cream Pie 235
Coconut Cake 256
Coconut Pound Cake 255

COFFEE CAKES
  Plantation Coffee Cake 119
  Poppyseed Coffee Cake 120
Coffee Punch 69
Colonial Cornbread 121
Colonial Pecan Pie 240
Company Chicken Divan 182
Company Eye of the Round 148
Company Meatloaf 153
Company Rice Casserole 219
Company Tuna 175
Congealed Asparagus Salad 97

COOKIES (Includes Bars and Squares)
  Applesauce Spice Squares 279
  Apricot Squares 278
  Blonde Brownies 273
  Boom Town Bliss Brownies 275
  Brickle Graham Bites 280
  Bumpy Brownies 273
  Butterscotch Brownies 274
  Butterscotch Cheesecake Bars 281
  Caramel Tennessee Bars 284
  Caroline's Chocolate Squares 278
  Chocolate Chip Oatmeal Cookies 266
  Cup Cake Brownies 274
  Date Crinkle Cookies 265
  Date Nut Bars 282
  Dixie Bars 280
  English Toffee Squares 282
  Fudge Brownie Bonbons 275
  Geneva's Brownies 277
  Kourabiedes (Greek Cookies) 266
  Lacy Cookies 272
  Lemon Crumb Cookies 267
  Lemon Dessert Squares 283
  Lemon Pecan Dainties 268
  Mint Chocolate Brownies 276
  Nana's Jelly Centers 268
  Nancy's Peanut Butter Cup Tarts 281
  Oatmeal Crunchies 269
  Pecan Shortbread Squares 284
  Pickwick Chocolate Chips 267

Praline Cookies 269
Presidential Brownies 277
Raspberry Kisses 270
Rocky Top Cookies 270
Sugar Cookies 271
Swiss Doubles 271
Three Way Cookies 272
Toffee Bars 283

CORN
  Corn Casserole 212
  Corn Chowder 77
  Corn Custard 211
  Corn Slaw 105
  Corn Soufflé 211
  Virginia's Corn Slaw 106

CORNBREAD
  Colonial Cornbread 121
  Corn Light Bread 121
  Corn Pones 121
  Cornbread Dressing 228
  Easy Cornbread 120
  Mexican Cornbread 122
Cornish Hen with Raspberry
  Sesame Sauce 188
Country Ham 158
Crab Pâté 52
Crab Rolls 52

CRABMEAT
  Cheesy Stuffed Potatoes 215
  Crab Pâté 52
  Crab Rolls 52
  Crabmeat Mornay 53
  Crabmeat Supreme in Coquille 166
  Deviled Crab 166
  Eggplant Supreme with Crabmeat 167
  Hot Crab Dip 62
  She-Crab Soup 82
  Southern Crab Dip 51

CRANBERRIES
  Ann's Cranberry Salad 89
  Chicken Cranberry Layer Salad 96
  Cranapple Crunch 295
  Cranberry Chutney 38
  Fresh Cranberry Sauce 226
  Pineapple Cranberry Punch 72
  Quick Cranberry Salad 98
Cream of Cucumber Soup 77
Cream Puffs 290
Creamy Broccoli Salad 104
Crème Vichyssoise 84
Creole Style Halibut 167
Croustades 39
Crunchy Vegetable Salad 109

CUCUMBERS
Cream of Cucumber Soup 77
Cucumber Cream Cheese Spread 37
Cucumber Mousse 37
Cucumber Salad 98
Cucumber-Onion in Marinade 107
Cup Cake Brownies 274

D

DATES
Chocolate Chip Date Cake 252
Date and Cheese Rolls 39
Date Crinkle Cookies 265
Date Nut Bars 282
Date Nut Loaf 127
David's Hollandaise Sauce 225
Delta Chocolate Pie 238
Delta Ice Cream 287

DESSERTS (See Cakes, Candy, Cookies and Pies)

Custards and Puddings
Brandied Caramel Flan 295
Bread Pudding/Lemon Sauce 293
Charlotte Russe 294
Cream Puffs 290
Flan 294
Four Step Pudding 297
Mom's Boiled Custard 293
No-Cook Banana Pudding 292
Peppermint Mousse 298

Frozen
Apricot Freeze 286
Baked Alaska 285
Banana Ice Cream 285
Chocolate Peppermints 287
Delta Ice Cream 287
Frozen Chocolate Mousse 286
Peach Ice Cream 289
Pineapple Sherbert 288
Ribbon Layered Lemon Pie 288
Tutti-Frutti Ice Cream 288
Vanilla Ice Cream 289

Fruit
Apple Crisp 291
Apple Kugel 291
Banana Split Dessert 292
Cranapple Crunch 295
Fresh Peach Soufflé 296
Fruit Pizza 296
Old Fashioned Strawberry
Shortcake 301
Orange Fig Whip 297
Raspberry Treat 298
Raspberry Trifle 299

Shortcake 290
Strawberries Jamaica 301
Strawberry Compote 300
Strawberry Lemon Dessert 301
Strawberry Soufflé 302
Deviled Crab 166
Deviled Eggs and Ham 198
Deviled Eggs with Mushrooms 197
Dieter's Spinach Quiche 202

DILL
Ann's Dill Bread 134
Best Coffee Can Dill Bread 135
Dill Dip 61
Dip for a Crowd 61
Dixie Bars 280
Dolmathakia (Stuffed
Grapevine Leaves) 50
Dove Breasts Stroganoff 190
Dove Pie 189
Doy's French Dressing 113
Dried Lima Bean Soup 76
Duck and Dried Tomato Salad 94
Duck Gumbo 78
Duck with Wild Rice 190

E

Easy Chicken and Rice 181
Easy Chocolate Sauce 303
Easy Cornbread 120
Easy Five-Hour Beef Stew 151
Easy Milk Chocolate Frosting 304
Easy Monkey Bread 123
Easy Poppy Seed Dressing 113
Easy Shrimp Dip 63

EGGPLANT
Eggplant Parmesan 212
Eggplant Supreme 213
Eggplant Supreme with Crabmeat 167
Ratatouille A La Doy 218
Shrimp and Eggplant Casserole 173

EGGS
Asparagus Soufflé 205
Bacon Quiche 202
Cheese Soufflé 199
Deviled Eggs and Ham 198
Deviled Eggs with Mushrooms 197
Dieter's Spinach Quiche 202
Eggs Whitney 196
Favorite Brunch Casserole 197
Holiday Breakfast Casserole 196
Quiche Individual 57
Sausage Cheese Crescent Squares 200
Sausage Grits Casserole 200
Swiss Bacon Lorraine 57

Elegant Green Bean Casserole 206
Elegant Pâté 45
Enchilada Casserole 152
English Toffee Squares 282
Ever So Easy Fruitcake 256
Eye of Round Roast 149

F

Fancy Chicken Spread 46
Fast Fudge 261
Favorite Brunch Casserole 197
Favorite Cheesecake 249
Fire and Ice Tomatoes 108

FISH
　　Baked Salmon Steaks 169
　　Company Tuna 175
　　Creole Style Halibut 167
　　Grilled Catfish with Dijon Sauce 165
　　Holiday Salmon Dip 63
　　Mexican Tuna Dip 65
　　My Caviar Cheese Ball 42
　　Parmesan Catfish Fillets 165
　　Poached Salmon with
　　　　Dilled Hollandaise 168
　　Tuna Roll 65
　　Tuna Salad 100
Flan 294
Four Step Pudding 297
French 75 70
French Market Soup 79
French Silk Chocolate Pie 237
Fresh Apple Cake 245
Fresh Broccoli-Cauliflower Salad 103
Fresh Cranberry Sauce 226
Fresh Peach Soufflé 296
Fresh Strawberry Cake 259
Fresh Strawberry Pie 244
Fresh Vegetable Mousse 59
Fresh Vegetable Squares 58

FROSTINGS
　　Caramel Icing 304
　　Easy Milk Chocolate Frosting 304
　　Old Fashion Cocoa Frosting 304
Frosty Peach Salad 101
Frozen Chocolate Mousse 286
Frozen Fruit Basket 102
Frozen Grape Salad 101

FRUIT (See individual Fruit listings)
　　Ambrosia Congealed Salad 96
　　Ever So Easy Fruitcake 256
　　Frozen Fruit Basket 102
　　Fruit Dip 63
　　Fruit Pizza 296
　　Fruit Punch 70

Fruit Salad Delight 102
Fruit Salad with Banana Cream 88
Fruit Salad with Tropical Sauce 88
Fruity Cream Cheese Spread 144
Honey Baked Fruit 226
Honey Dressing for Fruit 112
Hot Fruit Compote 227
Hot Gingered Fruit 227
Mixed Fruit Deluxe 87
Polynesian Fruit Salad 100
Tutti-Frutti Ice Cream 288
Fudge Brownie Bonbons 275
Fudge Pie 236

G

GAME
　Dove
　　Dove Breasts Stroganoff 190
　　Dove Pie 189
　　Grilled Dove Breasts 39
　Duck
　　Duck and Dried Tomato Salad 94
　　Duck Gumbo 78
　　Duck with Wild Rice 190
　　Jim's Wild Duck 191
　　Quick and Easy Duck 191
　Quail
　　Smothered Quail 192
Garlic Cheese Grits 196
Gazpacho 79
Gazpacho Aspic 95
Geneva's Brownies 277
George Washington Stuffed Roast 150
German Chocolate Pound Cake 253
Giblet Gravy 193
Gladys Brinckerhoff's Beans 207
Gourmet Beef Tenderloin 148
Gourmet Chocolate Sauce 303

GRAPES
　　Dolmathakia (Stuffed Grapevine
　　　　Leaves) 50
　　Frozen Grape Salad 101
Grape Cluster 141

GREEN BEANS
　　Bean Bundles 206
　　Elegant Green Bean Casserole 206
　　Green Bean Finger Sandwiches 55
Grilled Catfish with Dijon Sauce 165
Grilled Dove Breasts 39
Guacamole Salad Bowl 91

H

Ham and Turkey Casserole 162
Ham and Vegetable Casserole 163

Ham Roll Ups 161
Harvest Apple Cake 246
Harvest Sheaf 140
Hash Brown Potato Casserole 199
Hawaiian Chicken Salad 87
Herb Vinaigrette Dressing 113
Holiday Breakfast Casserole 196
Holiday Punch 70
Holiday Salmon Dip 63
Holiday Sweet Potatoes 217
Honey Baked Fruit 226
Honey Dressing for Fruit 112
Horseradish Mold 40
Hot Bean Dip 61
Hot Chicken Salad I 182
Hot Chicken Salad II 183
Hot Crab Dip 62
Hot Fruit Compote 227
Hot Gingered Fruit 227
Hot Rum Punch 72
Hot Slaw 106
Hot Tennessee Dip 64
Howard McClain's Easy Pie 239

I

ICE CREAM
Banana Ice Cream 285
Delta Ice Cream 287
Peach Ice Cream 289
Tutti-Frutti Ice Cream 288
Vanilla Ice Cream 289
Iced Broccoli Soup 75
Impossible Coconut Pie 239
Italian Cream Cake 257
Italian Summer Salad 93
Italian Tomatoes 108

J

Jane's Green Pea Casserole 214
Jeanne Craddock's Rolls 132
Jim's Wild Duck 191
Joann's Broccoli Muffins 123

K

Kahlúa Pecan Pie 241
Karen's Chicken Soufflé 183
Kate's Cream Cheese Braids 129
Khashapuri 142
Kourabiedes (Greek Cookies) 266
Kum Bac Salad Dressing 112

L

Lacy Cookies 272

LAMB
Lamb Shanks Milanese 164
Roast Leg of Lamb 163
Lasagna Casserole 156
Layered Taco Dip 65

LEMONS
Aunt Dot's Lemon Carrots 209
Blueberry Lemon Tea Cake 127
Bread Pudding/Lemon Sauce 293
Lemon Crumb Cookies 267
Lemon Dessert Squares 283
Lemon Nut Bread 131
Lemon Nut Cake 257
Lemon Pecan Dainties 268
Lemonade Pie 240
Ribbon Layered Lemon Pie 288
Strawberry Lemon Dessert 301
Libby's French Pastry Log 130

LIMA BEANS
Dried Lima Bean Soup 76
Gladys Brinckerhoff's Beans 207
Lite Sun Tea 73
Louisiana Chicken Spaghetti
for a Crowd 184

M

Mallett's Brunswick Stew 80
Manicotti 155
Margaret's Granola 264
Marinated Eye of Round Roast 149
Marinated Vegetable Medley 109
Marinated Veggies 110
Mary Ann Ward's Barbecued Brisket 147
Mary T's Pound Cake 254
Mashed Potato Casserole 214
May Bowl Punch 71

**MEATS (See Beef, Pork, Lamb and
Veal listings)**

MEXICAN
Chicken Enchilada Casserole 178
Chili Relleno Bake 158
Enchilada Casserole 152
Gazpacho 79
Gazpacho Aspic 95
Guacamole Salad Bowl 91
Layered Taco Dip 65
Mexican Cornbread 122
Mexican Squash 220
Mexican Tuna Dip 65
South of the Border Salad 94
Spanish Rice 219
Taco Casserole 153
Taco Salad 95
Tamale Casserole 157

Mini Cheesecakes 250
Mini Reuben Sandwiches 56
Mint Chocolate Brownies 276
Mint Sauce for Lamb 194
Mint Tea 74
Mixed Fruit Deluxe 87
Mom's Boiled Custard 293
Mother's Cheese Wafers 44
Moussaka 154

MUFFINS
Joann's Broccoli Muffins 123
Oatmeal Muffins 124
Party Muffins 124
Piña Colada Muffins 124
Plum Muffins 125
Mulled Wine 74
Mushroom Turnovers 48
My Caviar Cheese Ball 42
My Sister's Potatoes 215

N
Nana's Jelly Centers 268
Nancy's Peanut Butter Cup Tarts 281
Nanny's Chicken Pot Pie 185
New Orleans Milk Punch 71
Nina's Clam Dip 62
No-Cook Banana Pudding 292

O
Oatmeal Crunchies 269
Oatmeal Muffins 124
O'Farrell's Chicken Stew 184
Okra, Pickled 230
Old Fashion Cocoa Frosting 304
Old Fashioned Potato Salad 103
Old Fashioned Strawberry
Shortcake 301

ONIONS
Cucumber-Onion in Marinade 107
Very Best Onion Soup 80

ORANGES
Orange Balls 263
Orange Fig Whip 297
Orange Molded Salad 99
Orange Salad 98
Orange Wine Sauce 195
Oven Swiss Steak 151

OYSTERS
Oyster Casserole 228
Oysters Rockefeller 53

P
Parmesan Catfish Fillets 165
Parmesan Chicken 185

Parmesan Shrimp au Gratin
with Sherry 172
Party Muffins 124
Party Pecans 59
Pasta Salad 110

PEAS
Jane's Green Pea Casserole 214
Snow Peas with Boursin 54

PEACHES
Betty's Spiced Peaches 229
Fresh Peach Soufflé 296
Frosty Peach Salad 101
Peach Ice Cream 289
Pickled Peach Salad 89
Southern Peach Pie 242
Peanut Butter Fingers 262

PEARS
Pear Chutney 229
Pickled Pears 229
Pecan Shortbread Squares 284
Pecan Tarts 241
Peppermint Mousse 298
Percolator Punch 72
Pickled Okra 230
Pickled Peach Salad 89
Pickled Pears 229
Pickled Shrimp 54
Pickwick Chocolate Chips 267

PIES
Angel Chocolate Pie 236
Apple Pie 233
Banana Cream Pie 234
Chocolate Chess Pie 237
Chocolate Fudge Pie 235
Cocoa Cream Pie 235
Colonial Pecan Pie 240
Delta Chocolate Pie 238
French Silk Chocolate Pie 237
Fresh Strawberry Pie 244
Fudge Pie 236
Howard McClain's Easy Pie 239
Impossible Coconut Pie 239
Kahlúa Pecan Pie 241
Lemonade Pie 240
Pecan Tarts 241
Pineapple Cream Cheese Pie 242
Pumpkin Pie 243
Ribbon Layered Lemon Pie 288
Sherry Pie 244
Soda Cracker Pie 243
Southern Chess Pie 234
Southern Peach Pie 242
Southern Sweet Chocolate Dessert 300

"Watch Your Weight"
    Chocolate Cream Pie 238
Pimento Cheese Ball 42
Piña Colada Muffins 124

PINEAPPLE
    Pineapple Cheese Ball 43
    Pineapple Cheese Casserole 230
    Pineapple Cranberry Punch 72
    Pineapple Cream Cheese Pie 242
    Pineapple Dressing 112
    Pineapple Fruit Freeze 101
    Pineapple Sherbert 288
    Pineapple Upside Down Cake 258
Plantation Cheese Ball 43
Plantation Coffee Cake 119
Plum Muffins 125
Poached Salmon with Dilled
    Hollandaise 168
Pocketbook Rolls 133
Polynesian Fruit Salad 100
Poppy Seed Dressing 113
Poppyseed Coffee Cake 120

PORK
    Apricot Stuffed Pork 159
    Bacon Quiche 202
    Country Ham 158
    Deviled Eggs and Ham 198
    Ham and Turkey Casserole 162
    Ham and Vegetable Casserole 163
    Ham Roll Ups 161
    Holiday Breakfast Casserole 196
    Pork Chops Supreme 159
    Pork Tenderloin 161
    Sausage Cheese Crescent Squares 200
    Sausage Grits Casserole 200
    Sausage Rice Casserole 201
    Sausage Stuffed Mushrooms 49
    Sausage Surprise 201
    Sausage Swirls 50
    Sweet and Sour Meatballs 48
    Sweet and Sour Pork 160
    Swiss Bacon Lorraine 57

POTATOES
    Cheesy Stuffed Potatoes 215
    Crème Vichyssoise 84
    Hash Brown Potato Casserole 199
    Mashed Potato Casserole 214
    My Sister's Potatoes 215
    Old Fashioned Potato Salad 103
    Super Duper Potatoes 216
Praline Cookies 269
Presidential Brownies 277
Pumpkin Pie 243

Q
Quiche Individual 57
Quick and Easy Chicken Delight 187
Quick and Easy Duck 191
Quick Cranberry Salad 98
Quick Pepper Steak 149

R
Rainbow Pasta Salad 111

RASPBERRIES
    Cornish Hen with Raspberry
      Sesame Sauce 188
    Raspberry Kisses 270
    Raspberry Salad 99
    Raspberry Sauce 303
    Raspberry Treat 298
    Raspberry Trifle 299
    Swiss Doubles 271
Ratatouille A La Doy 218
Remoulade Sauce 195
Ribbon Layered Lemon Pie 288

RICE AND PASTA
    Artichoke-Rice Salad 102
    Chicken and Rice Delight 177
    Company Rice Casserole 219
    Duck with Wild Rice 190
    Easy Chicken and Rice 181
    Lasagna Casserole 156
    Louisiana Chicken Spaghetti
      for a Crowd 184
    Pasta Salad 110
    Rainbow Pasta Salad 111
    Rice Stodge 218
    Rice with Pine Nuts 218
    Sausage Rice Casserole 201
    Seafood and Wild Rice Casserole 170
    Shrimp Creole and Rice 171
    Spanish Rice 219
    Stuffed Pasta Shells 157
    Tiny Ring Macaroni Salad 111
    Tortellini 216
Richglen's Cheddar Cheesecake
    with Strawberries 247
Roast Leg of Lamb 163
Roast Turkey 188
Rocky Road 263
Rocky Top Cookies 270
Rum Cake 258

S

SALAD DRESSINGS
    Doy's French Dressing 113
    Easy Poppy Seed Dressing 113
    Herb Vinaigrette Dressing 113

Honey Dressing for Fruit 112
Kum Bac Salad Dressing 112
Pineapple Dressing 112
Poppy Seed Dressing 113
Sesame Salad Dressing 114
Shrimp Salad Dressing 114
Tarragon Salad Dressing 114

SALADS
Fruit
Ambrosia Congealed Salad 96
Ann's Cranberry Salad 89
Avocado Mandarin Green Salad 92
Chicken Cranberry Layer Salad 96
Frosty Peach Salad 101
Frozen Fruit Basket 102
Frozen Grape Salad 101
Fruit Salad Delight 102
Fruit Salad with Banana Cream 88
Fruit Salad with Tropical Sauce 88
Guacamole Salad Bowl 91
Mixed Fruit Deluxe 87
Orange Molded Salad 99
Orange Salad 98
Pickled Peach Salad 89
Pineapple Fruit Freeze 101
Polynesian Fruit Salad 100
Quick Cranberry Salad 98
Raspberry Salad 99
Tart Cherry Salad Mold 97

Meat/Seafood
Chicken Cranberry Layer Salad 96
Duck and Dried Tomato Salad 94
Guacamole Salad Bowl 91
Hawaiian Chicken Salad 87
Shrimp Salad 87
South of the Border Salad 94
Taco Salad 95
Tiny Ring Macaroni Salad 111
Tuna Salad 100

Vegetable
Artichoke Lettuce Salad 90
Artichoke-Rice Salad 102
Broccoli Mold 108
Broccoli Oriental Salad 104
Caesar Salad 91
Calico Vegetable Salad 105
Charlemagne Salad 90
Congealed Asparagus Salad 97
Corn Slaw 105
Creamy Broccoli Salad 104
Crunchy Vegetable Salad 109
Cucumber Salad 98
Cucumber-Onion in Marinade 107
Duck and Dried Tomato Salad 94

Fire and Ice Tomatoes 108
Fresh Broccoli-Cauliflower Salad ... 103
Gazpacho Aspic 95
Hot Slaw 106
Italian Summer Salad 93
Italian Tomatoes 108
Marinated Vegetable Medley 109
Marinated Veggies 110
Old Fashioned Potato Salad 103
Pasta Salad 110
Rainbow Pasta Salad 111
Sauerkraut Salad 107
Savory Summer Salad 107
Seven Layer Salad 93
Spinach Layered Salad 92
Sweet and Sour Slaw 106
Tiny Ring Macaroni Salad 111
Virginia's Corn Slaw 106
Sally Lunn Bread 134
SANDWICHES
Asparagus Sandwiches 55
Green Bean Finger Sandwiches 55
Mini Reuben Sandwiches 56
Sauce for Marshall Field
Sandwich 195
Tea Sandwiches 56
Sangría 73
SAUCES
Dessert
Bread Pudding/Lemon Sauce 293
Easy Chocolate Sauce 303
Gourmet Chocolate Sauce 303
Raspberry Sauce 303
Game
Wild Game Sauce 194
Meat
Blender Béarnaise Sauce 192
Cindy's Marinara Sauce 194
Cornish Hen with Raspberry
Sesame Sauce 188
Fresh Cranberry Sauce 226
Giblet Gravy 193
Mint Sauce for Lamb 194
Orange Wine Sauce 195
Sauce for Marshall Field
Sandwich 195
Spicy-Spicy Mustard 193
Sweet and Sour Sauce 66
Tangy Dipping Sauce 66
Veal Scallops in
White Wine Sauce 164
Seafood
Grilled Catfish with Dijon Sauce 165
Orange Wine Sauce 195

Poached Salmon with
   Dilled Hollandaise 168
   Remoulade Sauce 195

Vegetable
   David's Hollandaise Sauce 225
Sauerkraut Salad 107
Sausage Cheese Crescent Squares 200
Sausage Grits Casserole 200
Sausage Rice Casserole 201
Sausage Stuffed Mushrooms 49
Sausage Surprise 201
Sausage Swirls 50
Savory Summer Salad 107
Savory Vegetable Soup 84
Scalloped Broccoli Casserole 209

SEAFOOD
   Seafood and Wild Rice Casserole 170
   Seafood Bisque 81
   Seafood Casserole Royale 169
   Seafood Gumbo 81
Seasoned Oyster Crackers 59
Sesame Cheese Straws 44
Sesame Chicken Strips 47
Sesame Salad Dressing 114
Seven Layer Salad 93
She-Crab Soup 82
Sherry Pie 244
Shortcake 290

SHRIMP
   Easy Shrimp Dip 63
   Parmesan Shrimp au Gratin
      with Sherry 172
   Pickled Shrimp 54
   Shrimp and Eggplant Casserole 173
   Shrimp Creole 170
   Shrimp Creole and Rice 171
   Shrimp in Lemon Butter 171
   Shrimp Salad 87
   Shrimp Salad Dressing 114
   Shrimp Tomato Mold 51
   Shrimp Victoria 175
   Shrimp, Mushroom and
      Artichoke Casserole 174
   Southwest Shrimp Casserole 174
Skedaddles 264
Smothered Quail 192
Snow Peas with Boursin 54
Soda Cracker Pie 243

SOUPS
   Asparagus Soup 75
   Bonnie's Vegetable Soup 83
   Cheese Soup 76
   Clear Tomato Soup 83
   Corn Chowder 77
   Cream of Cucumber Soup 77
   Crème Vichyssoise 84
   Dried Lima Bean Soup 76
   Duck Gumbo 78
   French Market Soup 79
   Gazpacho 79
   Iced Broccoli Soup 75
   Mallett's Brunswick Stew 80
   Savory Vegetable Soup 84
   Seafood Bisque 81
   Seafood Gumbo 81
   She-Crab Soup 82
   Squash Soup 82
   Swiss Broccoli Soup 75
   Very Best Onion Soup 80
Sour Dough Bread 138
South of the Border Salad 94
Southern Chess Pie 234
Southern Crab Dip 51
Southern Dream Cake 259
Southern Fried Chicken 186
Southern Peach Pie 242
Southern Sweet Chocolate Dessert 300
Southwest Shrimp Casserole 174
Spanish Rice 219
Spicy Beets 208
Spicy-Spicy Mustard 193

SPINACH
   Dieter's Spinach Quiche 202
   Spinach Appetizers 58
   Spinach Layered Salad 92
   Spinach Madeleine 222
   Spinach New Orleans 222
   Spinach Supreme 223
Spoon Bread 122

SQUASH
   Mexican Squash 220
   Squash and Apple Bake 221
   Squash Soup 82
   Thanksgiving Squash 221
Steamed Buns 143
Steamed Zucchini 224

STRAWBERRIES
   Fresh Strawberry Cake 259
   Fresh Strawberry Pie 244
   Old Fashioned Strawberry
      Shortcake 301
   Richglen's Cheddar Cheesecake
      with Strawberries 247
   Strawberries Jamaica 301
   Strawberry Butter 144
   Strawberry Compote 300
   Strawberry Lemon Dessert 301
   Strawberry Punch 73

Index

Strawberry Soufflé 302
Stuffed Bread 144
Stuffed Cornish Hens with
   Apple Dressing 187
Stuffed Mushrooms 49
Stuffed Pasta Shells 157
Stuffed Tomatoes Houston Style 224
Sugar Cookies 271
Summer Vegetable Medley 220
Super Duper Potatoes 216
Sweet and Sour Chicken 186
Sweet and Sour Meatballs 48
Sweet and Sour Pork 160
Sweet and Sour Sauce 66
Sweet and Sour Slaw 106
Sweet Nothings 263

SWEET POTATOES
   Holiday Sweet Potatoes 217
   Sweet Potato Casserole 217
Swiss Bacon Lorraine 57
Swiss Broccoli Soup 75
Swiss Doubles 271

T
Taco Casserole 153
Taco Salad 95
Tamale Casserole 157
Tangy Dipping Sauce 66
Tarragon Salad Dressing 114
Tart Cherry Salad Mold 97
Tea Sandwiches 56
Tennis Tea 74
Thanksgiving Squash 221
Three Way Cookies 272
Tiny Ring Macaroni Salad 111
Tiropetakia (Cheese Puffs) 40
Toffee Bars 283

TOMATOES
   Baked Herb Tomatoes 223
   Clear Tomato Soup 83
   Duck and Dried Tomato Salad 94
   Fire and Ice Tomatoes 108
   Italian Tomatoes 108
   Shrimp Tomato Mold 51
   Stuffed Tomatoes Houston Style 224

Tomato Soup Dip 64
Tortellini 216
Tuna Roll 65
Tuna Salad 100
TURKEY
   Ham and Turkey Casserole 162
   Roast Turkey 188
Tutti-Frutti Ice Cream 288

U
Uncle Henry's Milk Punch 71

V
Vanilla Ice Cream 289
Vanilla Wafer Cake 255
Veal Scallops in White Wine Sauce 164
**VEGETABLES (See individual
   Vegetable listings)**
   Antipasto 35
   Bonnie's Vegetable Soup 83
   Buffet Mixed Vegetables 213
   Calico Vegetable Salad 105
   Crunchy Vegetable Salad 109
   Fresh Vegetable Mousse 59
   Fresh Vegetable Squares 58
   Gazpacho 79
   Gazpacho Aspic 95
   Ham and Vegetable Casserole 163
   Marinated Vegetable Medley 109
   Marinated Veggies 110
   Savory Vegetable Soup 84
   Summer Vegetable Medley 220
Very Best Onion Soup 80
Virginia's Corn Slaw 106

W
"Watch Your Weight"
   Chocolate Cream Pie 238
Whole Wheat Bread 139
Wild Game Sauce 194

Z
Zucchini, Steamed 224

Auxiliary to the Memphis Dental Society
P. O. Box 17272
Memphis, Tennessee 38187-0272

Please send me _____copies of *Impressions*   @ $16.95 each _____
Tennessee residents add 7¾% sales tax   @   1.31 each _____
Postage and handling   @   2.50 each _____
Gift wrap   @   1.00 each _____
                                                        Total Enclosed _____

Name _____

Address _____

City _____ State _____ Zip _____

Make checks payable to *Impressions*.
All proceeds will be used for dental health projects.

- -

Auxiliary to the Memphis Dental Society
P. O. Box 17272
Memphis, Tennessee 38187-0272

Please send me _____copies of *Impressions*   @ $16.95 each _____
Tennessee residents add 7¾% sales tax   @   1.31 each _____
Postage and handling   @   2.50 each _____
Gift wrap   @   1.00 each _____
                                                        Total Enclosed _____

Name _____

Address _____

City _____ State _____ Zip _____

Make checks payable to *Impressions*.
All proceeds will be used for dental health projects.

- -

Auxiliary to the Memphis Dental Society
P. O. Box 17272
Memphis, Tennessee 38187-0272

Please send me _____copies of *Impressions*   @ $16.95 each _____
Tennessee residents add 7¾% sales tax   @   1.31 each _____
Postage and handling   @   2.50 each _____
Gift wrap   @   1.00 each _____
                                                        Total Enclosed _____

Name _____

Address _____

City _____ State _____ Zip _____

Make checks payable to *Impressions*.
All proceeds will be used for dental health projects.

- -

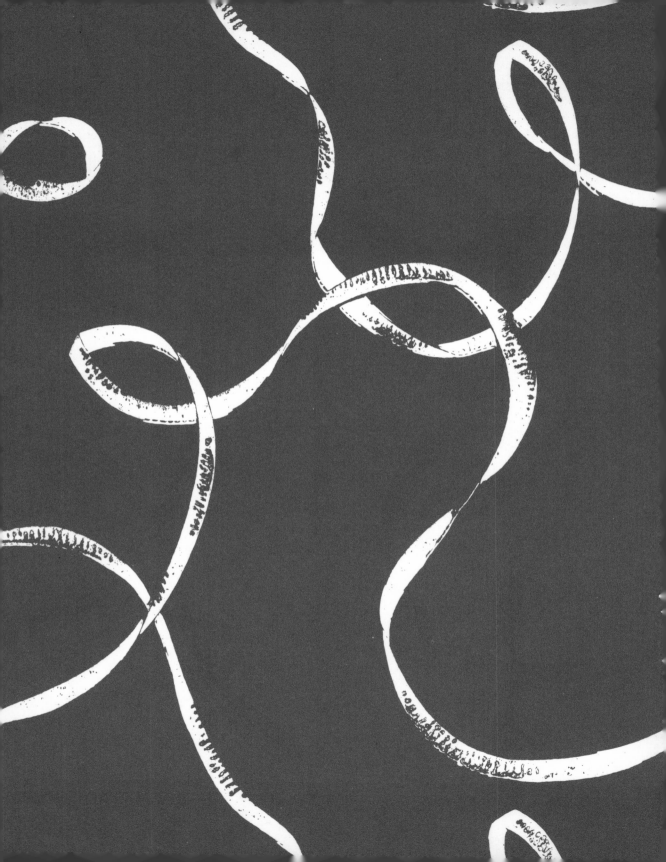